# The Johns Hopkins Handbook of In Vitro Fertilization and Assisted Reproductive Technologies

# The Johns Hopkins Handbook of In Vitro Fertilization and Assisted Reproductive Technologies

Edited by

**Marian D. Damewood, M.D.**
Associate Professor of Gynecology and Obstetrics, Division of Reproductive
Endocrinology, Director of In Vitro Fertilization Program, Johns Hopkins
University School of Medicine, Baltimore, Maryland

**Little, Brown and Company**
**Boston/Toronto/London**

Copyright © 1990 by Marian D. Damewood

First Edition

Library of Congress Catalog Card No. 90-060733

ISBN 0–316–17194–8

Printed in the United States of America

RRD-VA

To Rick and Diana

# Contents

**Contributing Authors**

**Preface**

**I. PRE—IVF-ET SCREENING**

1. **Selection of Patients for In Vitro Fertilization—Embryo Transfer**    3
   Eugene Katz and Bradley S. Hurst

2. **Andrologic Parameters for IVF-ET**    14
   Bradley S. Hurst and William D. Schlaff

3. **Psychological Issues in IVF: Evaluation and Care**    27
   Peter J. Fagan and Yula Ponticas

**II. THE IVF-ET TEAM**

4. **Personnel and the Organization of the IVF Team**    39
   Marian D. Damewood and Sharon G. Meng

5. **IVF Office Procedure**    43
   Marian D. Damewood and Teresa M. Zemanski

6. **Informed Consent for IVF Procedures**    51
   Marian D. Damewood

**III. THE IVF-ET PROCEDURE**

7. **Physiologic Principles of Induction of Ovulation**    61
   Howard A. Zacur and Arnold Goodman

8. **Follicular Maturation and Monitoring for IVF-ET**    69
   John S. Hesla

9. **Techniques of Oocyte Retrieval**    92
   Bruce L. Tjaden and John A. Rock

**IV. LABORATORY**

10. **Laboratory Preparation for Human IVF-ET**    103
    Meriella J. Hubbard and Leslie Weikert

11. **Morphology of Unfertilized and Fertilized Oocytes**    114
    Meriella J. Hubbard and Leslie Weikert

**V. CONTEMPORARY PROCEDURES ASSOCIATED WITH IVF-ET**

12. **Gamete Intrafallopian Transfer: Current Perspectives**    125
    Ricardo Azziz

13. **Cryopreservation in a Human IVF Program**    142
    Lynette Wilson

**VI. CURRENT CONSIDERATIONS IN ASSISTED REPRODUCTIVE TECHNOLOGIES**

14. **Ethical Aspects of IVF and Related Assisted Reproductive Technologies**    151
    Edward E. Wallach

15. **IVF Financial Considerations**    163
    Marian D. Damewood and Edward E. Wallach

**Index**    177

# Contributing Authors

**Marian D. Damewood, M.D., Editor**
Associate Professor of Gynecology and Obstetrics, Division of Reproductive Endocrinology, Director of In Vitro Fertilization Program, Johns Hopkins University School of Medicine, Baltimore, Maryland

**Ricardo Azziz, M.D.**
Assistant Professor, University of Alabama School of Medicine; Department of Obstetrics and Gynecology, Division of Reproductive Endocrinology, University of Alabama Hospital, Birmingham, Alabama

**Peter J. Fagan, Ph.D.**
Assistant Professor of Medical Psychology and Psychiatry, Johns Hopkins University School of Medicine; Director of Sexual Behaviors Consultation Unit, Johns Hopkins Hospital, Baltimore, Maryland

**Arnold Goodman, Ph.D.**
Associate Professor of Gynecology and Obstetrics and Physiology, Johns Hopkins University School of Medicine, Baltimore, Maryland

**John S. Hesla, M.D.**
Assistant Professor of Gynecology and Obstetrics, Division of Reproductive Endocrinology, Johns Hopkins University School of Medicine; Director, Section of Reproductive Surgery, Johns Hopkins Hospital, Baltimore, Maryland

**Meriella J. Hubbard, M.S., M.A.S.**
Instructor of Gynecology and Obstetrics, Johns Hopkins University School of Medicine; Senior Embryologist, In Vitro Fertilization Laboratory, Division of Reproductive Endocrinology, Johns Hopkins Hospital, Baltimore, Maryland

**Bradley S. Hurst, M.D.**
Instructor of Gynecology and Obstetrics, Johns Hopkins University School of Medicine; Division of Reproductive Endocrinology, Johns Hopkins Hospital, Baltimore, Maryland

**Eugene Katz, M.D.**
Assistant Professor of Gynecology and Obstetrics, University of Maryland School of Medicine; Director, In Vitro Fertilization Program, University Hospital, Baltimore, Maryland

**Sharon G. Meng, R.N.C., B.S.N., M.P.H.**
Nurse Coordinator, In Vitro Fertilization Program, Department of Gynecology and Obstetrics, Johns Hopkins University School of Medicine; Division of Reproductive Endocrinology, Johns Hopkins Hospital, Baltimore, Maryland

**Yula Ponticas, Ph.D.**
Instructor of Medical Psychology and Psychiatry, Johns Hopkins University School of Medicine; Sexual Behaviors Consultation Unit, Johns Hopkins Hospital, Baltimore, Maryland

**John A. Rock, M.D.**
Professor of Gynecology and Obstetrics, Johns Hopkins University School of Medicine; Director, Division of Reproductive Endocrinology, Johns Hopkins Hospital, Baltimore, Maryland

**William D. Schlaff, M.D.**
Associate Professor of Gynecology and Obstetrics, University of Colorado School of Medicine; Director, Division of Reproductive Endocrinology, University of Colorado Hospital, Denver, Colorado

**Bruce L. Tjaden, D.O.**
Instructor of Gynecology and Obstetrics, Johns Hopkins University School of Medicine; Division of Reproductive Endocrinology, Johns Hopkins Hospital, Baltimore, Maryland

**Edward E. Wallach, M.D.**
Professor of Gynecology and Obstetrics, Division of Reproductive Endocrinology, Johns Hopkins University School of Medicine; Director of Gynecology and Obstetrics, Johns Hopkins Hospital, Baltimore, Maryland

**Leslie Weikert, B.S.**
Department of Gynecology and Obstetrics, Johns Hopkins University School of Medicine; Embryologist, In Vitro Fertilization Laboratory, Division of Reproductive Endocrinology, Johns Hopkins Hospital, Baltimore, Maryland

**Lynette Wilson, M.S.**
Embryologist, Department of Gynecology and Obstetrics, Arlington Hospital, Arlington, Virginia

**Howard A. Zacur, M.D., Ph.D.**
Associate Professor and Deputy Director of Gynecology and Obstetrics, Johns Hopkins University School of Medicine; Division of Reproductive Endocrinology, Johns Hopkins Hospital, Baltimore, Maryland

**Teresa M. Zemanski**
Administrative Secretary, Department of Gynecology and Obstetrics, Johns Hopkins University School of Medicine; Division of Reproductive Endocrinology, Johns Hopkins Hospital, Baltimore, Maryland

# Preface

Since the first successful human in vitro fertilization in 1978, culminating in the birth of Louise Brown in the United Kingdom, in vitro technology has been associated with far-reaching implications in the field of human reproduction. Investigations of previously uncharted areas of human gamete function, fertilization, and early embryonic development have been undertaken. Cryopreservation techniques for embryos, once limited to animal husbandry, have been successfully applied to the human conceptus. Alternate forms of reproduction such as gamete intrafallopian transfer have developed as corollary procedures of the in vitro fertilization process. In addition, the scientific advances associated with human in vitro fertilization have generated profound ethical issues associated with manipulation of the fertilized human oocyte. The use of donor gametes, the use of a surrogate uterus, and the possibility of blastocyst manipulation and sperm microinjection have raised issues important to scientific, clerical, and governmental leaders.

The first human in vitro fertilization procedure was performed by laparoscopic retrieval techniques in a natural cycle resulting in the fertilization of one oocyte. Present day technology includes control of the hypothalamic pituitary axis with GnRH analogs and induction of ovulation with human menopausal gonadotropins resulting in the development of multiple follicles. Oocyte retrieval techniques have been modified to include an ultrasound directed vaginal retrieval approach. Sperm microinjection techniques, as well as new cryopreservative techniques for embryos, sperm, and oocytes, are under investigation.

Of utmost importance in the organization of successful IVF programs is the team approach to these procedures. The participation of a team of physicians, laboratory staff, nursing staff, anesthesiology, and laboratory medicine have all contributed to successful in vitro outcomes. It is uncommon in medicine, with the exception of transplantation teams, to have such a comprehensive team approach to a procedure—an approach that has contributed markedly to the innovative scientific advances and the success of this new reproductive technology.

M.D.D.

# The Johns Hopkins Handbook of In Vitro Fertilization and Assisted Reproductive Technologies

# Pre–IVF-ET Screening

# Selection of Patients for In Vitro Fertilization–Embryo Transfer

Eugene Katz and Bradley S. Hurst

The first successful extracorporeal fertilization and cleavage of a human egg is that of Rock and Menkin in 1944 (34). Thirty years later the extracorporeal fertilization of a human egg and cleavage to the blastocyst stage in vitro with subsequent transfer of the fertilized donor egg to a recipient's uterus was reported (39). The culmination of extracorporeal fertilization of a human egg was the birth of Louise Brown when Edwards and Steptoe successfully completed an in vitro fertilization with an embryo transfer (IVF-ET) in 1978. One earlier attempt resulted in an ectopic pregnancy (41).

The publicity generated by the birth of a "test-tube" baby produced a host of requests to the medical community for the IVF-ET procedure. In the early years of IVF-ET, women with tubal disease who were not considered candidates for established therapies became the primary candidates for this procedure; however, as the success rates, costs, and risks of IVF-ET became more clearly defined, the criteria for patient selection have been expanded to include patients with other causes of infertility (Table 1-1).

Before pursuing IVF-ET a complete infertility evaluation is mandatory. More established and traditional therapies also should be considered given the success rates, expenses, and relative risks involved with IVF-ET. A national IVF pregnancy rate of 16% per cycle (27) coupled with the high costs involved with each attempt must be compared with the success, expense, and risks involved with traditional therapies. This chapter reviews the major indications for the IVF-ET procedure and the traditional therapies in an effort to establish guidelines for patient selection.

## TUBAL DISEASE

Microsurgical techniques were introduced in infertility surgery to enhance the prognosis, especially in the correction of tubal and adhesive peritoneal disease. The microsurgical lysis of extra-adnexal adhesions, salpingolysis, fimbrioplasty, salpingostomy, tubotubal anastomosis, and tubouterine implantation were the immediate applications for the patient with tubal infertility.

Pregnancy rates following tubal surgery depend on the type of procedure selected, the condition of the tube, and the experience of the surgeon. The presence of peritubular adhesions, the condition of the tubal muscular wall, the ciliary epithelium, and the degree of fimbrial damage also affect the outcome following microsurgical tubal reconstruction and repair (35). Large hydrosalpinges of more than 3 cm, absence of fimbria, and severe adhesions are associated with a poor prognosis following surgery (Table 1-2). Patients undergoing salpingostomy for distal tubal obstruction are unlikely to achieve a full-term live-birth pregnancy. Recent reports demonstrate a live-birth rate of between 20–30% with an additional 20% experiencing an ectopic pregnancy when the data were assembled using life table analysis (18, 19).

Patients who remain infertile following a tuboplasty are unlikely to conceive following a second procedure, especially when followed by a salpingostomy (20) (Figure 1-1). Repeat surgery may be indicated in patients with tubes in good condition and with minimal adhesions. Surgery can enhance the IVF-ET attempt by making the ovaries accessible for vaginal or laparoscopic retrieval.

The prognosis following a tubal reanastomosis varies according to the type of sterilization procedure, the site of anastomosis, and the tubal length on com-

**Table 1-1. Causes of infertility in patients in the Johns Hopkins IVF-GIFT program**

| Major causes of infertility | Percentage of total | |
|---|---|---|
| | IVF | GIFT |
| Tubal disease | 39.2 | — |
| Endometriosis (stages I–IV) | 25.8 | 43.2 (stages I–II) |
| Unexplained infertility | 23.6 | 39.8 |
| Oligospermia | 6.2 | 5.6 |
| Immunologic factors | 3.1 | 10.3 |
| Cervical factor | 2.1 | 1.1 |

**Table 1-2. Pregnancy outcome and tubal patency following salpingostomy**

| Extent of disease | Pregnancy outcome (%) | Ectopic pregnancies (%) | Postoperative hysterogram patency (%) |
|---|---|---|---|
| Mild | 86 | 6 | 100 |
| Moderate | 26 | 12 | 74 |
| Severe | 8 | 2 | 65 |

Source: K.S. Moghissi, Unexplained infertility. *Fertil. Steril.* 39:5, 1983.

pletion of the procedure. Poor outcomes are associated with monopolar cautery sterilization and tubes less than 4 cm in length. The outcome is dismal for patients who have undergone fimbriectomy. Pregnancy rates reported range from as high as 50% with uterotubal reimplantation to 8% or less with concomitant severe adhesive disease.

Repeated ectopic pregnancy is an indication for IVF. The risk of a third ectopic pregnancy after two conservative interventions remains high whereas 30% of women may achieve an intrauterine pregnancy (7).

IVF pregnancy success rates for patients with tubal disease are comparable to those of patients with other factors or causes undergoing IVF, or both (Table 1-3). Oocyte recovery is less for patients with reduced ovarian access although the severity of periovarian adhesions does not appear to impair follicular development (8). Patients with bilateral tubal ligation have significantly higher pregnancy rates per cycle and per transfer than patients with severe ovarian disease. The overall pregnancy rates achieved for each group, however, are not significantly different from those patients with tubal factor (32).

When the pregnancy rate one expects to achieve falls below 20% following surgical therapy in patients with tubal infertility, IVF-ET is the option suggested to couples for consideration. Patients who remain infertile following tubal surgery and patients who wish to bypass surgical therapy may elect for IVF-ET. Since it has been shown that with ovarian access extensive adhesive disease does not appear to affect IVF-ET success rates and that prior adnexal surgery has no known effect on IVF-ET outcome, adhesiolysis is not a prerequisite to IVF-ET.

Success rates vary significantly from one IVF program to another. Recent data from Oehninger and colleagues (32) demonstrated a 22% pregnancy rate per cycle in 1031 IVF-ET cycles from 549 patients with tubal infertility. Most programs fail to achieve a 20% success rate with IVF as indicated by recent data from the United States National IVF Registry (27). National statistics, however, are not directly applicable to all IVF programs.

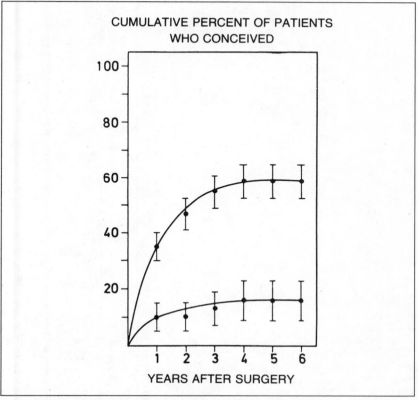

Fig. 1-1. Cumulative conception rates for 102 cases undergoing tubal surgery. The lower graph represents the group of patients treated with repeated tuboplasties. The upper represents the group undergoing a single tuboplasty. The vertical bars show the standard error for the proportion of pregnant patients. (From J. G. Lauritzen et al. Results of repeated tubuloplasties. *Fertil. Steril.* 37:68, 1982. With permission.)

Couples with tubal infertility should be advised to consider IVF-ET as an option when the expected pregnancy rate is below 20% following surgery. Patients with failed surgical therapy or patients for whom surgery is not an option may elect IVF in place of surgery. As suggested, extensive adhesions do not significantly lower the chance of success with IVF-ET as long as the ovaries are accessible. Prior adnexal surgery has no effect on IVF-ET outcome (32). Adhesiolysis is therefore not necessary prior to IVF as long as ovaries are accessible for retrieval.

## ENDOMETRIOSIS

The association of endometriosis and infertility is well known, although the pathophysiologic mechanism responsible for the failure to conceive remains uncertain. An analysis of the possible effects of the ectopic endometrial tissue or of the influence of the environment that allowed the reimplantation or development of such tissue is beyond the scope of this chapter. Poor folliculogenesis, luteal phase defect, hyperprolactinemia, luteinized unruptured follicle syndrome, autoimmune factors, mechanical factors, increased peritoneal prosta-

Table 1-3. Pregnancy rates versus diagnosis in the IVF program in Norfolk

| Diagnosis | Patients | Cycles | Transfers | Pregnancies | Pregnancies per cycle (%) | Pregnancies per transfer (%) |
|---|---|---|---|---|---|---|
| Tubal disease | 266 | 478 | 377 | 89 | 18.6 | 24 |
| Endometriosis | 11 | 20 | 15 | 6 | 30 | 40 |
| Male factor | 23 | 30 | 11 | 3 | 10 | 27 |
| Normal infertile | 11 | 18 | 13 | 5 | 28 | 38 |
| Miscellaneous | 8 | 14 | 13 | 2 | 14 | 15 |
| Total | 319 | 560 | 429 | 105 | 18.8 | 24.5 |

Source: P.G. Wardle et al. *Lancet* 2(46):552, 1985.

**Table 1-4. Pregnancy success with various therapeutic modalities for patients with endometriosis**

| Therapy | Mild | Moderate | Severe |
|---|---|---|---|
| **Crude pregnancy rates*** | | | |
| Traditional therapies | | | |
| Expectant management [38] | 92/183 (50) | — | — |
| Danazol [38] | 205/511 (40) | 52/132 (39) | 31/78 (40) |
| $CO_2$ laser laparoscopy [25] | 387/682 (57) | 208/420 (50) | 45/90 (50) |
| Conservative resection [36] | 28/45  (62) | 44/88  (55) | 33/66 (50) |
| **Pregnancies per cycle*** | | | |
| Assisted reproductive technologies | | | |
| Superovulation [9] | | | |
| (with IUI) | 12/65  (18) | 4/23  (17) | 0/5 |
| | | (includes all | |
| GIFT [38] | 10/43  (23) | stages) | |
| | | | (moderate and |
| IVF-ET [31] | 46/191 (24.1) | 7/35  (20) | severe) |

*Percentages within parentheses.

glandins, and macrophages have all been associated with endometriosis and infertility (17).

Therapeutic alternatives for endometriosis include expectant management, medical therapy, surgical therapy, and assisted reproductive technologies.

In cases of minimal and mild disease, there is little evidence to suggest that medical or surgical intervention is better than observation alone (33) (Table 1-4). In patients with severe disease, up to 50% conceive following surgery (25, 36). Assisted reproductive technologies including superovulation with intra-uterine insemination (IUI) and gamete intrafallopian transfer (GIFT) are associated with pregnancy rates per cycle of 18% (9) and 23% (38), respectively, although normal tubal anatomy is necessary for both.

IVF is an alternative for the patient with endometriosis and pelvic adhesions or tubal disease and in those who remain infertile following traditional therapeutic approaches.

Reports of success vary among IVF treatment centers. Recent data from the Norfolk program reported a per cycle pregnancy rate of 22% in 136 patients undergoing 280 IVF cycles compared to tubal factor control group of 22.3% (31). Patients with minimal and mild endometriosis showed no significant difference in the stimulation response, fertilization rate, luteal phase progesterone, or pregnancy rates per transfer. Significantly, more oocytes were recovered in patients with American Fertility Society stages I and II disease. Other studies have shown evidence of lower fertilization rates in vitro in patients with endometriosis (45, 49). Some authors attribute a lower pregnancy rate per transfer to poor quality conceptus or defective luteal phase in severe endometriosis (4). The clinical significance of these subtle abnormalities is unclear. With IVF-ET, patients with all stages of endometriosis have pregnancy rates comparable to other groups undergoing IVF. Patients with mild disease seem to have better pregnancy rates than other groups (4, 46) (Table 1-3).

## MALE FACTOR

IVF and ET are logical alternatives for oligospermic men. Because sperm are placed in direct contact with oocyte, a relatively low concentration of sperm is adequate for fertilization. Fertilization rates, although lower in oligospermic men, are acceptable with sperm densities above $1.5 \times 10^6$ per ml after swim-up (44).

Oligospermia is often associated with poor motility. Many laboratory techniques have been developed to concentrate motile sperm for use in IVF. Optimum fertilization of an oocyte is achieved with the use of $0.5-2.0 \times 10^5$ motile sperm per ml in oligospermic men (47). Once fertilization occurs, pregnancy rates per transfer are as good as or better than normospermic groups (15).

Due to lower fertilization rates, pregnancy rates may be expected to be lower with male infertility (Table 1-3). Results with IUIs are initially equal (14) but better in the long term (1) than IVF. Comparisons of IVF and GIFT for the treatment of male factor infertility show comparable success (22), although GIFT provides no data on the fertilizing capacity of the sperm in unsuccessful cycles. IVF followed by tubal embryo transfer or zygote intrafallopian transfer represents a compromise between the last two options (50). Fertilized eggs are allowed to continue their development in the more natural environment, the fallopian tube, allowing a better-timed and gentler arrival into the uterine cavity. When alternative therapies for abnormal semen parameters fail, IVF-ET, tubal embryo transfer, or GIFT becomes an option providing that an adequate number of motile sperm can be recovered after semen processing.

## CERVICAL FACTOR

It was initially suggested that couples with poor postcoital tests have lower fertilization rates than patients with tubal or unexplained infertility (16). This finding is not universally accepted (26).

If the cervical mucus cannot be improved medically, IUIs should be performed to bypass the cervix. Bypassing the cervix is a less expensive and simple alternative for patients with cervical factor due to a local mucus problem (1). Only after an unsuccessful trial period of therapy should IVF-ET become an alternative.

## IMMUNOLOGIC FACTOR

The presence of antisperm antibodies in either the female or the male can interfere with the process of conception. In the female, antisperm antibodies have been detected in the plasma, genital tract, and follicular fluid. In males, antisperm antibodies can be present in plasma and semen (2).

Immunosuppression, condoms, and periodic abstinence have been used to reduce the levels of antibodies. Success, however, has been limited and side effects of immunosuppression unacceptable.

IVF-ET is successful in overcoming infertility due to immunologic factors (5, 6, 33, 48), although patient numbers have been small and diagnostic tests employed and therapies vary considerably in the literature. IVF should be considered when other therapeutic measures have failed.

## IDIOPATHIC INFERTILITY

The term *idiopathic,* or unexplained infertility, is applied to couples who have failed to conceive after 2 years of regular intercourse and in whom no definitive pathology or anomaly of the reproductive systems can be identified. It may also be used to denote patients who remain infertile after the etiologic factors are identified and have undergone therapy. Unexplained infertility is present in 15% of all infertile couples (28).

It is important to consider the natural history of couples with unexplained infertility before proceeding with any form of therapy. Unfortunately, even in recent studies, many patients have been labeled "idiopathic" without having undergone a diagnostic laparoscopy. It is estimated that 5% of women under 30 years of age with unexplained infertility will become pregnant each subsequent year (23). After 7 years, 36.2% of the couples presenting with primary idiopathic

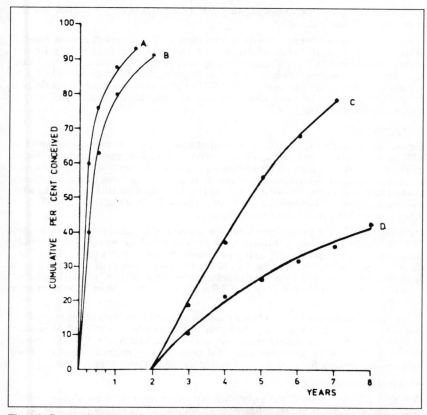

Fig. 1-2. Conception rates of a normal population of parous (A) and nulliparous (B) women are compared with the cumulative conception rates of apparently normal women with secondary infertility (C) and primary infertility (D). No conceptions occurred before the 2- to 3-year interval in the infertile groups as this was part of the selection criteria for these patients. (From E. A. Lenton et al. Long term follow-up of the apparently normal couple with a complaint of infertility. *Fertil. Steril.* 28:913, 1977. With permission.)

infertility conceive (Fig. 1-2). Management of couples with unexplained infertility is directed at improving cycle fecundity when expectant management is rejected by the couple, the physician, or both. IUIs, Pergonal, and Pergonal combined with IUIs increase pregnancy rates per cycle to 2.7% (40), 6.1% (40), and 19% (9), respectively, for couples with unexplained infertility.

Success rates with GIFT (19% per attempt) and IVF (20% per attempt) have been shown to be comparable in couples with idiopathic infertility in a prospective study by Lenton and colleagues (22).

IVF can bypass subtle defects in ovulation, ovum pick-up, gamete transport, and tubal environment that may be present in couples with unexplained infertility. IVF provides documentation of fertilization. Abnormal oocytes can be identified. Careful observation of sperm morphology in patients with unexplained fertilization failure in vitro has provided the basis for a stricter criteria to evaluate defects in sperm morphology (30). IVF, therefore, may provide insight to the "occult" male factor.

Patients with unexplained infertility who elect IVF can expect results comparable to patients with tubal infertility and endometriosis (Table 1-3). Recent reports comparing IVF fertilization rates, conception rates, miscarriage rates, and viable pregnancy rates have shown no significant difference when comparing unexplained infertility to controls (29). Couples with secondary unexplained infertility appear to be more likely to achieve pregnancies than couples with primary infertility (24).

## PATIENT AGE

Tieze (42) calculated that 11% of women at age 34 were infertile, compared to 33% at age 40 and 87% at age 44. A study of women undergoing artificial insemination with frozen donor semen due to absolute male sterility showed a significant decline in fertility and cumulative pregnancy rates in the 31–35 age group and again in the 36–40 age group (11). The rapid decline in fertility with advancing age often reduces the observation period before electing IVF-ET after other therapies have been attempted.

Data regarding IVF pregnancy rates for women with advancing age are conflicting (Table 1-5). Data published by Wilkes and colleagues (46) from Norfolk showing improved pregnancy rates in women between the ages of 36–40 are disputed by more recent studies. Gianaroli and colleagues (13) demonstrated a decline in IVF pregnancies with advancing patient age, with a "take-home baby" rate of 4.6% per oocyte recovery and 5.7% per embryo transfer in women over 38.

These data should not be used to exclude women over 38 from attempting IVF. A strong argument can be made, however, for proceeding to IVF-ET in women in their younger years rather than saving IVF as a last resort. Couples should be counseled as to the maternal and fetal risks during pregnancy and the need for prenatal testing for chromosome disorders should pregnancy occur.

## OVARIAN DISORDERS

IVF and ET can benefit patients with hypogonadotropic anovulation, oligo-ovulation, and luteal phase deficiency, although IVF is rarely indicated when these disorders exist as isolated conditions. IVF or GIFT is still the procedure of choice in patients with luteinized unruptured follicle syndrome. Polycystic ovarian disease has been suggested as indication for IVF-ET by some authors (37). IVF may decrease the risk of hyperstimulation and the multiple pregnancy rate seen with gonadotropin therapy in polycystic ovarian patients, although IVF does not eliminate these risks (37).

IVF-ET has provided a means for achieving a pregnancy in menopausal patients due to premature ovarian failure, oophorectomy gonadal dysgenesis, or patients with resistant ovary syndrome through the use of donor oocytes. Successful pregnancies have been reported following IVF of donor oocytes (3, 12, 13, 21). Many ethical and legal issues remain unresolved or untested and include the legal status of a child resulting from a donor oocyte procedure, donor confidentiality, and the selection and screening of oocyte donors. These issues must be clearly understood and accepted by the patients, donors, and IVF program before electing to proceed with donor oocytes.

## GENETIC DISORDERS

Donor oocytes are used in women with genetic disease to avoid passing the disease to their offspring. Donor oocyte use has been reported in patients with Turner's syndrome, 46 × 0/XX mosaics, 47 XXX, and in a patient with Huntington's chorea (3). Obviously, the use of donor oocytes does not eliminate the possibility of genetic or nongenetic congenital defects.

Table 1-5. Pregnancies per cycle

| Age | Wilkes | Gianaroli |
|---|---|---|
| 20–30 | 27/138 (19.6%) | |
| 22–29 | | 30/136 (22.1%) |
| 30–34 | | 31/250 (12.4%) |
| 31–35 | 46/303 (15.2%) | |
| 36–40 | 32/188 (27.1%) | |
| >38 | | 6/132 (4.5%) |

Source: C. A. Wilkes et al. Pregnancy related to infertility diagnosis, number of attempts, and age in a program of in vitro fertilization. *Obstet. Gynecol.* 66:350, 1985, and L. Gianaroli et al. The role of the patient's age in the outcome of IVF cycles. *Hum. Reprod.* 3 (Suppl. 1), Aug. 1988.

Advanced biochemical and genetic techniques may one day allow for the diagnosis of genetic disease in preimplantation embryos. Currently, experimental typing of spermatozoa for the presence of X or Y chromosomes may be feasible. Embryos may be assessed by evaluating metabolite uptake, products produced by the embryo, or by enzyme assays. DNA probes also may prove useful to evaluate specific chromosomes for genes in the preimplantation embryo (10).

## UTERINE DISEASE

Patients with müllerian agenesis, congenital uterine anomalies, and women with severe intrauterine adhesions refractory to surgical lysis of the adhesions as well as hysterectomized patients can, through IVF, transfer their embryos to a surrogate mother (43). Legal and ethical issues for surrogate mothers are complex and remain unsolved.

## CONCLUSIONS

IVF-ET is an option for an increasing number of couples with infertility. The indications for IVF reviewed in this chapter will surely change as IVF-ET technology continues to improve. All therapeutic options should be presented to the couple, and treatment should be individualized based on the etiology of infertility, patient age, and the expected success with each option. Unfortunately, cost and insurance coverage remain a major deciding factor for many. Although IVF-ET is no longer considered a "last resort" treatment, IVF provides hope for many when other options have failed.

## REFERENCES

1. Allen, N.C., et al. Intrauterine insemination: A critical review. *Fertil. Steril.* 44:569, 1986.
2. Bronson, R., Cooper, G., and Rosenfield, D. Sperm antibodies: Their role in infertility. *Fertil. Steril.* 42:171, 1984.
3. Chan, C.L.K., et al. Oocyte donation and in vitro fertilization for hypergonadotropic hypergonadism: Clinical state of the art. *Obstet. Gynecol. Surv.* 42:350, 1987.
4. Chillik, C.F., et al. The role of in vitro fertilization in infertile patients with endometriosis. *Fertil. Steril.* 44:56, 1985.
5. Clarke, G.N., et al. Effect of sperm AB in males in human IVF. *Am J. Reprod. Immunol. Microbiol.* 8:62, 1985.
6. Clarke, G.N., et al. In vitro fertilization results for women with sperm antibodies in plasma and follicular fluid. *Am J. Reprod. Immunol. Microbiol.* 8:130, 1985.
7. DeCherney, A.H., et al. Reproductive outcome following two ectopic pregnancies. *Fertil. Steril.* 43:82, 1985.
8. Diamond, M.P., et al. The effect of periovarian adhesions on follicular development in patients undergoing ovarian stimulation for in vitro fertilization-embryo transfer. *Fertil. Steril.* 49:100, 1988.

9. Dodson, W.C., et al. Superovulation with intrauterine insemination in the treatment of infertility: A possible alternative to gamete intrafallopian transfer and in vitro fertilization. *Fertil. Steril.* 48:441, 1987.
10. Edwards, R.G., and Hollands, P. New advances in human embryology: Implications of the preimplantation diagnosis of genetic disease. *Hum. Reprod.* 3:549, 1988.
11. Federation CECOS, Schwartz, D., and Mayaux, M.J. Female fecundity as a function of age. Results of artificial insemination in 2193 nulliparous women with azoospermic husbands. *N. Engl. J. Med.* 306:404, 1982.
12. Feichtinger, W., and Kemeter, P. Pregnancy after total ovariectomy achieved by ovum donation. *Lancet* 2(8457):722, 1985.
13. Gianaroli, L., et al. The role of the patient's age in the outcome of IVF cycles. *Hum. Reprod.* 3(Suppl.) 1:83, 1988.
14. Hewitt, J., et al. Treatment of idiopathic infertility, cervical mucus hostility, and male infertility: Artificial insemination with husband's semen or in vitro fertilization? *Fertil. Steril.* 44:350, 1985.
15. Hirsch, I., et al. In vitro fertilization in couples with male factor infertility. *Fertil. Steril.* 45:659, 1986.
16. Hull, M.G.R., et al. An economical and ethical way to introduce in vitro fertilization to infertility practice, and findings related to post coital sperm/mucus penetration in isolated tubal, "cervical" and unexplained infertility. *Ann. N.Y. Acad. Sci.* 442:318, 1985.
17. Hurst, B.S., and Rock, J.A. Endometriosis: Pathophysiology, diagnosis and treatment. *Obstet. Gynecol. Surv.* 44(5):293, 1989.
18. Jacobs, L.A., et al. Primary microsurgery for post-inflammatory tubal infertility. *Fertil. Steril.* 50:855, 1988.
19. Laotikainen, T.J., et al. Factors influencing the success of microsurgery for distal tubal occlusion. *Arch. Gynecol. Obstet.* 243:101, 1988.
20. Lauritzen, J.G., et al. Results of repeated tuboplasties. *Fertil. Steril.* 37:68, 1982.
21. Leeton, J., et al. A controlled study between the use of gamete intrafallopian transfer (GIFT) and in vitro fertilization-embryo transfer in the management of idiopathic and male infertility. *Fertil. Steril.* 48:605, 1987.
22. Lenton, E.A., Weston, G.A., and Cooke, I.D. Long term follow-up of the apparently normal couple with a complaint of infertility. *Fertil. Steril.* 28:913, 1977.
23. Lessing, J.B., et al. The performance of primary and secondary unexplained infertility in an in vitro fertilization-embryo transfer program. *Fertil. Steril.* 50:903, 1988.
24. Lutjen, P., et al. The establishment and maintenance of pregnancy using in vitro fertilization and embryo donation in a patient with primary ovarian failure. *Nature* 307:174, 1984.
25. Martin, D.C., and Rock J.A. Endoscopic surgical treatment of endometriosis. Presented at the George W. Mitchell International Colloquium, San Antonio, October 29, 1988.
26. Matson, P.L., et al. The value of the postcoital test in predicting the fertilization of human oocytes. *J. In Vitro Fert. Embryo Transf.* 3:110, 1986.
27. Medical Research International and the Society of Assisted Reproductive Technology, The American Fertility Society. In vitro fertilization/embryo transfer in the United States: 1987 results from the National IVF-ET Registry. *Fertil. Steril.* 51:13, 1989.
28. Moghissi, K.S., and Wallach, E.E. Unexplained infertility. *Fertil. Steril.* 39:5, 1983.
29. Navot, M.D., et al. The value of in vitro fertilization for the treatment of unexplained infertility. *Fertil. Steril.* 49:854, 1988.
30. Oehninger, S., et al. Failure of fertilization in in vitro fertilization: The "occult" male factor. *J. In Vitro Fert. Embryo Transf.* 5:181, 1988.
31. Oehninger, S., et al. In vitro fertilization and embryo transfer (IVF/ET): An established and successful therapy for endometriosis. *J. In Vitro Fert. Embryo Transf.* 5:249, 1988.

32. Oehninger, S., et al. Effects of the severity of tubo-ovarian disease and previous tubal surgery on the results of in vitro fertilization and embryo transfer. *Fertil. Steril.* 51:126, 1989.

33. Potashnik, G., et al. Results of in vitro fertilization in women with antisperm antibodies in serum, cervical mucus, and follicular fluid. *J. In Vitro Fert. Embryo Transf.* 5:199, 1988.

34. Rock, J., and Menkin, M.F. In vitro fertilization and cleavage of human ovarian eggs. *Science* 100:105, 1944.

35. Rock, J.A., et al. Factors influencing the success of salpingostomy techniques for distal fimbrial obstruction. *Obstet. Gynecol.* 52:591, 1978.

36. Rock, J.A., et al. The conservative surgical treatment of endometriosis: Evaluation of pregnancy success with respect to the extent of disease as categorized using contemporary classification systems. *Fertil. Steril.* 35:131, 1981.

37. Salat-Baroux, J., et al. Results of IVF in the treatment of polycystic ovary disease. *Hum. Reprod.* 3:331, 1988.

38. Schenken, R.S. (ed.). *Endometriosis: Contemporary Concepts in Clinical Management.* Philadelphia: Lippincott, 1989.

39. Schumacher, G.F.B., et al. In vitro fertilization of human ova and blastocyst transfer—An invitational symposium. *J. Reprod. Med.* 11:192, 1973.

40. Serhal, P.F., et al. Unexplained infertility—the value of Pergonal superovulation combined with intrauterine insemination. *Fertil. Steril.* 49:602, 1988.

41. Steptoe, P. Historical aspects of the ethics of in-vitro fertilization. *Ann. N.Y. Acad. Sci.* 442:602, 1988.

42. Tieze, C. Reproductive span and rate of reproduction among Hutterite women. *Fertil. Steril.* 8:89, 1957.

43. Utian, W.H., et al. Successful pregnancy after in vitro fertilization and embryo transfer from an infertile woman to a surrogate. *N. Eng. J. Med.* 313:1251, 1985.

44. Van Uem, J.F.H.M., et al. Male factor evaluation in in vitro fertilization: Norfolk experience. *Fertil. Steril.* 44:375, 1985.

45. Wardle, P.G., et al. Endometriosis and ovulatory disorders: Reduced fertilization in-vitro compared with tubal and unexplained infertility. *Lancet* 2(8454):552, 1985.

46. Wilkes, C.A., et al. Pregnancy related to infertility diagnosis, number of attempts, and age in a program of in vitro fertilization. *Obstet. Gynecol.* 66:350, 1985.

47. Wolf, D.O. Semen assessment in IVF. *J. In Vitro Fert. Embryo Transf.* 3:341, 1986.

48. Yovich, J.L., et al. In vitro fertilization of oocytes from women with serious antisperm antibodies. *Lancet* 1(8373):369, 1984.

49. Yovich, J.L, et al. In vitro fertilization for endometriosis. *Lancet* 2(8454):552, 1985.

50. Yovich, J.L., et al. Pregnancies following pronuclear stage tubal transfer (PROST). *Fertil. Steril.* 48:851, 1987.

# Andrologic Parameters for IVF-ET

Bradley S. Hurst and William D. Schlaff

In vitro fertilization (IVF) has provided new insights into the etiology and treatment of male factor infertility (3). IVF allows direct evidence of sperm fertilizing capacity compared to prior standards including semen analysis, postcoital testing, sperm penetration assay (SPA), and other methods used in the past from which function was inferred. IVF enhances the possibility of fertilization by increasing the direct interaction of sperm and oocytes with relatively low concentrations of sperm. For many couples with male factor infertility, IVF represents the best chance for fertility short of donor insemination; however, results for these couples have been disappointing in many instances. Proper identification of couples likely to benefit from IVF is necessary to help couples decide whether IVF is the right choice for them.

Male factor infertility must be evaluated thoroughly. If other associated infertility factors are identified, treatment should be strongly considered before attempting IVF. This chapter deals with evaluation and treatment of male factor infertility by IVF.

## MALE INFERTILITY—DIAGNOSIS

Evaluation of the male is an essential aspect in the evaluation of an infertile couple and includes history, physical exam, and laboratory findings. Although commonly overlooked, a directed history from the husband can often give insight to problems and modify therapeutic options. Prior paternity is encouraging unless other problems have since arisen; however, one should not be deluded into thinking that a man with poor sperm parameters who has previously fathered children has developed a new problem. Prior reproductive success may be affected in great part by the relative fertility potential of the female partner. History of exposure to toxic substances, chemotherapy, irradiation, extreme heat or cold, or extreme stress represent problems that can have a profound impact on spermatogenesis. History or current evidence of a urinary tract infection, urgency, frequency, dysuria, penile discharge, or lesions may indicate a treatable infectious process.

Mumps orchitis, testicular trauma such as rupture or biopsy, or vasectomy reversal may result in oligospermia and sperm antibody production. Low sex drive or coital infrequency due to male disinterest may indicate an abnormal hormonal factor including hypogonadism or hyperprolactinemia. A personal or family history of birth defects, recurrent abortions, or family history of infertility raises the possibility of male chromosome anomalies.

Physical exam may indicate systemic illnesses that may lower the count. The penis should be examined for hypospadias or epispadias. The testes should be palpated and measured. The presence of a varicocele should be noted. Rectal exam with prostate massage can be performed to evaluate for prostatitis.

## DIAGNOSTIC METHODS

Laboratory tests are necessary to determine treatment and prognosis prior to initiating IVF. Although many diagnostic procedures and tests have been used to evaluate male fertility potential, laboratory diagnosis begins with semen analysis (Table 2-1). To give an adequate profile of male parameters, two to three semen analyses should be obtained.

Men with reduced semen parameters should be investigated further. Serum luteinizing hormone (LH), follicle stimulating hormone (FSH), testosterone (T), and prolactin should be measured. If gonadotropins and T are low, the patient

**Table 2-1. World Health Organization criteria for normal semen analysis**

| | |
|---|---|
| Volume | 2.0 ml or more |
| pH | 7.2–7.8 |
| Sperm concentration | $20 \times 10^6$ spermatozoa per ml or more |
| Total sperm count | $40 \times 10^6$ spermatozoa or more |
| Motility | 50% or more with forward progression or 25% or more with rapid linear progression within 60 min after collection |
| Morphology | 50% or more with normal morphology |
| Viability | 50% or more live, i.e., excluding dye |
| White blood cells | Fewer than $1 \times 10^6$ per ml |
| Zinc (total) | 2.4 μmol or more per ejaculate |
| Citric acid (total) | 52 mol (10 mg) or more per ejaculate |
| Fructose (total) | 13 μmol or more per ejaculate |

Source: World Health Organization. *Laboratory Manual for the Examination of Human Semen and Semen-Cervical Mucus Interaction.* Cambridge: Cambridge University Press, 1987.

should be evaluated for a central hypothalamic-pituitary defect. Such defects could possibly be treated hormonally. If gonadotropins are elevated and T is low or low normal, gonadal failure is likely, particularly if the testes are small. In such a case, the semen parameters are unlikely to improve even with therapy. Most commonly, oligospermic men will have normal LH and T and normal or slightly elevated FSH. Elevated FSH is a function of seminiferous epithelial dysfunction, and the associated decrease in inhibin secretion and loss of negative feedback centrally. Testes may be normal in size or slightly small. In either case, no medical therapy has been identified that will predictably enhance sperm parameters. Assisted forms of reproduction and particularly IVF may be the best option for these couples if donor insemination is not acceptable.

A most significant finding is azoospermia in association with normal hormone values and normal-sized testes. One must assume that this is secondary to obstruction. Such an obstruction may be either congenital or acquired due to surgery, infection, or injury. Seminal fructose, which is derived from the seminal vesicles, should be measured. Absence of fructose in the ejaculate implies obstruction distal to the seminal vesicles. This is one of the relatively few circumstances in which testicular biopsy may be indicated. Biopsy may be coupled with a vasogram or exploratory surgery depending on the findings.

Leukocytes in the semen at a concentration greater than $1 \times 10^6$ per ml should be further investigated. The patient should be closely examined for evidence of prostatitis or other genital tract infection. A semen culture for chlamydia, aerobic and anaerobic bacteria, and possibly mycoplasma and ureaplasma should be performed. Even if no infectious organism is identified, empiric treatment should be considered due to the known deleterious effect of leukocytes on fertilization (31).

Although the cervical mucus is bypassed by IVF, a postcoital test can be useful to further define abnormalities of sperm function. Poor sperm movement despite good cervical mucus suggests the presence of sperm antibodies. Antibody-bound sperm are frequently described as shaking in place or completely immotile. Sperm antibodies are much more common in men (90%) compared to women. Sperm antibodies may interfere with fertilization directly by binding to the sperm head or less directly by decreasing function though tail binding. In fact, antibodies are bound most commonly to both head and tail. Sperm antibody binding is also suggested by poor sperm motility in the face of normal sperm concentration at the time of a routine semen analysis. Finally, men who have previously had vasectomies are at high risk for having antibodies, particularly if the procedure was performed 10 or more years previously.

Sperm antibodies have traditionally been diagnosed by the sperm immobilization (Isojima) test or a variety of sperm agglutination (Kibrick, Franklin-Dukes) tests (17). These are indirect tests performed on patient serum mixed with donor sperm. More recently the sperm immunobead test has been utilized (6). Rabbit anti-human immunoglobulins are conjugated to microscopically visible polyacrylamide beads, which will then bind to sperm antibodies. The advantages of this test are that both direct and indirect assays can be performed, and that location and gross quantification of antibody binding can be observed. Although there is still controversy over the level of binding that should be considered significant, a figure of 20% is most commonly used.

The zona-free hamster test (egg penetration test, hamster test) is frequently touted as the most predictive test of sperm-fertilizing capacity. This test will be considered thoroughly in a later section.

## TREATMENT

Conditions should be optimal for the husband before moving on to IVF. Patients should be removed from toxic exposure, and stressful situations should be reduced if possible. If recent illness has lowered counts, IVF should be delayed. Infections should be treated appropriately as determined by culture and sensitivity results. Patients with hypogonadotropic hypogonadism should be treated with Pergonal or pulsatile gonadotropin releasing hormone as indicated. Hyperprolactinemic patients should be adequately suppressed with bromocriptine, and hypothyroid patients should receive adequate replacement. Azoospermic males who are hormonally normal with normal testes deserve further detailed urologic evaluation, since surgery can be effective in some cases of obstruction. Patients with significant antibody factors may improve with prednisone, 40 mg on days 1–7 of the spouse's menstrual cycle.

Finally, not to be forgotten, is donor insemination. In the absence of other female factors, donor insemination is a very safe and effective way to treat male factor infertility.

## IVF FOR MALE INFERTILITY

After the aforementioned measures are taken, IVF is a consideration. IVF has been used in cases of oligospermia, asthenospermia, teratospermia antisperm antibodies, and unexplained infertility.

### Oligospermia

Since IVF requires relatively few sperm for fertilization, oligospermic patients would seem to be ideal candidates for the procedure. A completely specific and sensitive technique for prospectively identifying those oligospermic men whose sperm will successfully fertilize the eggs of their wives is obviously highly desirable. Unfortunately, none has been found. Alternately, one could screen on the basis of the number of sperm alone, but no universally accepted minimal sperm concentration for IVF success exists. This is in part due to the absence of standard techniques for sperm preparation for IVF, so results may vary among centers as a function of laboratory methods. This problem is further confounded by the wide variation in function that can be seen in association with oligospermia. Oligospermia rarely exists as an isolated problem, and studies that lump patients with "male factor" infertility including oligospermia, asthenospermia, and teratospermia may result in data that are difficult to interpret. Finally most data in the literature are retrospective and not well controlled.

Given the limitations in the existing data, recurring trends are evident in the literature. Fertilization rates are consistently lower in oligospermic versus normospermic males (10, 18, 23, 33, 35, 39) (Table 2-2). Despite lower fertilization

**Table 2-2. Sperm concentration and fertilization in oligospermic couples**

| Study | Sperm concentration × $10^6$ per ml | Fertilization rate (%) | (controls) | Pregnancy rate (%) | (controls) |
|---|---|---|---|---|---|
| Van Uem et al. [33] | < 1.5* | Rare | (89) | | |
| Yovich and Stanger [39] | < 5* | 48 | (85) | | |
| Margalioth et al. [28] | 2–10 | 43 | | | |
| Mahadevan, Trounson, and Leeton [25] | < 10 | 25 | | | |
| Yovich and Stanger [39] | 6–11.5* | 77 | (85) | | |
| Junk et al. [18] | < 12* | 44 | (78) | | |
| Margalioth et al. [28] | 10–20 | 40 | | | |
| Mahadevan, Trounson, and Leeton [25] | 10–20 | 54 | | | |
| Leeton et al. [23] | < 20 | 42 | (65) | | |
| Wolf et al. [35] | < 20 | 49 | (76) | 28.5 | (20) |
| Diamond et al. [10] | < 20 | 52.9 | (65) | | |
| Van Uem et al. [33] | < 20 | 39.6 | (89) | 31 | (23) |

*Motile sperm per ml.

rates, oocytes are still fertilized frequently with sperm densities above $1.5 \times 10^6$ sperm per ml after separation (33). Once fertilization occurs and embryos are transferred, pregnancy rates per cycle are as good as (16) or better than normospermic groups (7, 23, 39). The offspring of oligospermic couples who conceive through IVF do not appear to have an increased risk of fetal anomalies as had once been feared (33).

One cannot explain lowered fertilization with oligospermic samples based on lowered concentrations alone. Several centers have examined fertilization by the same number of motile sperm in oligospermic and normospermic males (10, 33, 35) (Table 2-3). Despite controlling for concentration and motility, oligospermic males are less efficient at fertilizing oocytes than are normospermic males. Lowered motility, abnormal morphology, or other factors may play a role in this lowered fertilizing ability. Oligospermic men tend to have more favorable fertilization rates at higher fertilizing concentrations than their normal counterparts. Thus, although normal men fertilize oocytes quite well with concentrations of 50,000 per ml per oocyte (35), fertilization is improved in oligospermic men by using higher concentrations (500,000 per ml per oocyte) (10, 35).

Unfortunately, severely oligospermic men may be unable to achieve concentrations of 500,000 motile cells after preparation. Thus, severely oligospermic men may not be able to improve fertilization rates by using higher sperm concentrations in the lab preparation. Some centers choose to inseminate more than one oocyte per dish using a higher concentration of sperm in an attempt to overcome this problem.

Although severely oligospermic patients can expect a significant enhancement in fertilization with IVF, one must assess the likelihood of success with low numbers and seek to establish an absolute threshold below which success is effectively nil. In 1981, Craft and colleagues (9) reported successful fertilization in vitro with only 10,000 motile sperm in the culture fluid containing an oocyte. In 1985, Cohen and colleagues (7) reported seven pregnancies resulting from men with less than $0.5 \times 10^6$ per ml motile sperm in 15 patients. One embryo was replaced in at least 80% of patients, and 43.7% (7/16) achieved pregnancy (7); however, Van Uem and colleagues (33) in Norfolk achieved fertilization in only one patient when a motile sperm number less than $1.5 \times 10^6$ was used with multiple oocytes per dish. Variability in results from these centers makes it difficult to establish a minimal effective concentration of motile sperm that can be used for IVF; however, IVF for severely oligospermic males should only be attempted in centers with excellent fertilization rates and considerable experience in dealing with oligospermic samples to provide the couple maximum benefit.

### Asthenospermia

Studies evaluating the prognostic potential for IVF with asthenospermia suffer the same limitations as discussed for oligospermia and other individual seminal parameters. Decreased motility is uncommonly an isolated factor, and thus it is difficult to exclude the confounding factors of oligospermia and abnormal sperm morphology.

Wolf and colleagues (35) have shown a marked decrease in oocyte fertilization with sperm motility less than 40%. Other investigators have shown a decreased fertilization efficiency with motility less than 30% (16). Mahadevan and Trounson (24) noted decreased fertilization rates when initial motility was 30–49%. There was a further decrease in fertilization with motility between 20–29% and no fertilization when the initial motility was less than 20%. After semen preparation, no fertilization was reported for motility less than 30%. Despite this correlation, patients with low motility alone were noted to have a 56.8% fertilization rate compared to 20.8% when asthenospermia was combined with oligospermia or abnormal morphology (35). Cohen (7) similarly showed that

**Table 2-3. Sperm concentrations for insemination in oligospermic couples**

| Study | Motile sperm concentration per egg (number per ml) | Normal fertilization oligospermic | | Normospermic controls (%) |
|---|---|---|---|---|
| Van Uem et al. [33] | 100,000 | 45.5% | (5/11) | |
| | 100,000–490,000 | 55.0% | (11/20) | |
| | 500,000–790,000 | 47.9% | (23/48) | |
| Wolf et al. [35] | 50–100,000 | 30.7% | (4/13) | (61–75) |
| | 500,000 | 61.5% | (16/26) | (60) |
| Diamond et al. [10] | 250,000 | 48% | (12/25) | (67.9) |
| | 375,000 | 59% | (23/34) | (66.7) |
| | 500,000 | 84.7% | (11/13) | (58.7) |

fertilization did not decrease in samples with less than 20% motility or progression less than grade 2 until the motile sperm count fell below $2 \times 10^6$ per ml. Despite these reports, Edwards and colleagues (12) have reported fertilization with motility less than 10%. Fertilization failed in 60% of oocytes in combined oligoasthenospermia. The variability in data makes it difficult to establish motility criteria for acceptance into IVF programs; however, in general, couples with motility less than 30% can expect lowered fertilization, and IVF should be discouraged if motility is less than 10%.

## Abnormal Morphology

Sperm morphology is another factor that may affect fertilization in vitro; however, reports in the literature vary widely with some investigators suggesting no role and others suggesting morphology as an important factor.

Hirsch and colleagues (16) showed no statistically significant relationship between fertilization in vitro and abnormal sperm morphology when abnormal morphology was defined as greater than 40% abnormal forms. Mahadevan and Trounson (24) demonstrated a fertilization rate of 66.7% when abnormal morphology was an isolated finding. When associated with oligospermia or low motility, fertilization fell to 25%.

Yovich and Stanger (39) described delayed fertilization with abnormal morphology of greater than 60%. Fewer oocytes reached the pronuclear stage by 6–12 hours when there was a high percentage of morphologically abnormal sperm. The number of developing embryos was not significantly different from controls by 44–48 hours. Fertilization tended to be delayed more when head defects were present compared to tail defects. Patient numbers were too small to show significance.

Kruger and colleagues (21) proposed the use of stricter criteria for morphology than usual. To be considered normal, their criteria included an oval smooth head, 5–6 um in length and 2.5–3.5 um in width. No cytoplasmic droplets could be greater than 50% of the size of the head, and the acrosome must compose 40–70% of the head. Finally, there could be no head, midpiece, or tail defects. Borderline forms according to this system are considered abnormal. Using these criteria, these investigators found the fertilization rate to be 37% if less than 14% of sperm were morphologically normal compared to 81% if 15–30% of sperm were normal (20). Their studies imply that the standard World Health Organization criteria for abnormal morphology (37) may not be clinically useful in predicting IVF success. Severely abnormal morphology, at least by the criteria proposed by Kruger and colleagues, may be useful in screening for the suitability of a husband for IVF, but more studies are necessary to be conclusive.

## Autoimmunity

Approximately 5–10% of men have autoimmunity to sperm (15). Antisperm antibodies may interfere with cumulus dispersal, sperm binding to the zona pellucida, sperm penetration through the zona, or fertilization (34). Meaningful data regarding prognosis for IVF are limited, however, due the variability in tests used to detect sperm antibodies, small numbers of patients studied, and variability of sperm preparation techniques.

Cohen and colleagues (7) described IVF for men with autoantibodies assessed by the gelatin or tray agglutination tests or the mixed antiglobulin reaction, or a combination. Autoimmunity was diagnosed after antibodies were found in serum or seminal plasma on at least two separate occasions. Using these criteria, fertilization occurred in six out of seven couples, each undergoing one IVF attempt. Two pregnancies were achieved. These data suggest a favorable outcome; however, other studies have shown a poor correlation between antifertilization effects and the gelatin and tray agglutination tests (11).

Immunobeads can be used to test for IgA, IgG, and IgM antisperm antibodies on motile sperm. When couples with endometriosis, female sperm antibodies, or abnormal sperm morphology were excluded, fertilization (30%) was significantly lower when IgA and IgG were both bound to motile sperm than fertilization (78%) when no antibodies were bound (18). The presence of either IgA or IgG antibodies alone did not lower fertilization rates that were 79% and 75%, respectively (18); however, the study size was too small to allow significant statistical analysis. Although fertilization rates are lower when IgA and IgG antibodies are present, fertilization has been observed when 100% of motile sperm are bound by IgA and IgG antibodies (25). As one would expect, the combination of IgA and IgG binding and oligospermia appears to be associated with lower fertilization rates; however, the data are, as yet, inadequate to demonstrate a statistically significant difference.

## LABORATORY EVALUATION AND PROGNOSIS

With standard semen parameters insufficient to predict those males likely to fertilize or fail to fertilize oocytes for IVF, laboratory tests with high predictive values are needed. Of these, the SPA has been the most widely investigated.

### Sperm Penetration Assay

Data in the literature have been confusing and contradictory since the first description generally attributed to Wolf, Sokoloski, and Quigley in 1983 (36), correlating the SPA and IVF. A recent review by Mao and Grimes (26) summarized the findings to date, relating the prognostic benefit of the SPA in IVF (Table 2-4).

Careful inspection of the data reveals some of the pitfalls in evaluating the predictive value for the SPA. Overall patient numbers were small. Studies were inconsistent with regard to the definition of normal and abnormal results. Rogers (30) and Foreman and colleagues (13) defined abnormal tests as the absence of sperm penetration. Wolf and colleagues (36), Van Uem and colleagues (33), and Rudak and colleagues (32) defined normal penetration as 10% or more. Ausmanas and colleagues (2) defined a penetration of less than 15% as abnormal, and Margalioth and colleagues (28) used less than 20% penetration as the lower limit for fertile sperm. With the large disagreement in the definition of an abnormal range, it is not surprising that a wide discrepancy exists between results obtained from one study to another.

Wolf and colleagues (36) and Rogers (30) performed the SPA at the time of IVF. Although this timing should more directly show the physiologic correlation between the SPA and human oocyte fertilization, their data did not demonstrate that the SPA was useful as a screening test prior to IVF. Timing of the SPA was variable or unstated with the other studies except that of Ausmanas and colleagues (2) who performed the assay within 2 weeks of the IVF attempt. In this study, the sensitivity, specificity, and predictive value of an abnormal test were decreased.

When individual studies are evaluated in more detail, the results are less conclusive than might otherwise be suspected. For example, in the study by Wolf and colleagues (36), when fertilization failure because of abnormal oocytes was excluded, all couples achieved fertilization. The comparison of normal and abnormal SPA tests is therefore meaningless for this study. In the study by Foreman and colleagues (13), 15 couples were selected into the study after they had failed to fertilize oocytes in a prior IVF attempt. This patient selection bias suggests that those who perform poorly with IVF are likely to have an abnormal SPA. The study, however, fails to conclusively demonstrate that those with an abnormal SPA are unlikely to fertilize.

The study by Margalioth and colleagues (28) found the SPA to be a poor predictor of outcomes in couples with male infertility, whereas Van Uem and colleagues

Table 2-4. Correlation of sperm penetration assay and IVF

| Authors | Number of patients | Abnormal range[a] | Abnormal SPA | | Normal SPA | | Time of assay |
|---|---|---|---|---|---|---|---|
| | | | No fertilization[b] | Fertilization[b] | No fertilization[b] | Fertilization[b] | |
| Wolf, Sokoloski, and Quigley [36] | 24 | <10 | 0 | 3 | 7 | 17 | At time of IVF |
| Rogers [30] | 29 | 0 | 2 | 2 | 2 | 23 | At time of IVF |
| Foreman et al. [13] | 37 | 0 | 10 | 1 | 19 | 42 | Not stated |
| Ausmans et al. [2] | 54 | <15 | 1 | 14 | 2 | 37 | Within 2 wk |
| Van Uem et al. [33] | 19 | <10 | 7 | 0 | 2 | 12 | Not stated |
| Margalioth et al. [27] | 134 | <20 | 21 | 6 | 16 | 91 | Variable |
| Rudak et al. [32] | 68 | <10 | 9 | 27 | 4 | 28 | Variable |

[a]Percentage of hamster eggs penetration.
[b]IVF cycles.

(33) obtained good correlation between the SPA and human oocyte fertilization. More recent reports in the literature have failed to clarify the usefulness of the SPA (2, 8, 21, 22).

Many explanations have been suggested for the poor reproducibility of results for the SPA in predicting human oocyte fertilization. SPA laboratory techniques have varied, and factors such as sperm preparation methods, media, sperm concentrations, incubation capacitation times, and lengths of abstinence can affect outcomes (26). Human oocyte fertilization may also depend on factors other than sperm quality, including ovulation induction, patient age, etiology of infertility, timing of human chorionic gonadotropin, oocyte retrieval, and IVF laboratory procedures (32). Furthermore, SPA and human IVF involve different functions. The SPA evaluates the ability of the sperm to undergo capacitation and the acrosome reaction; fertilization requires a number of other functions including zona binding. The human oocyte is left intact for IVF, whereas the hamster egg is treated enzymatically prior to the SPA. The zona pellucida or cumulus cells, or both, may aid in sperm function and capacitation (22). With the conflicting reports in the literature and the cost for the SPA, which is rarely paid by insurers, the performance of the SPA as a screening procedure for IVF must be justified by data described in individual centers.

The hemizona assay (HZA) has been investigated as another means to predict the fertilizing potential of spermatozoa. Unlike the SPA, the HZA evaluates sperm binding to the human zona pellucida. The HZA is performed by cutting a human oocyte in half using a micromanipulation knife. Sperm is then coincubated with the hemizonae and assessed for sperm binding (5).

In a study evaluating the HZA, sperm from fertile men exhibited significantly higher binding capacity to hemizonae (34 ± 8.1 bound) compared with sperm from men with male factor infertility who had failed to fertilize their wives' oocytes on one or more IVF attempt (5.9 ± 2.3 bound). Due to the limited test numbers in the study, a threshold for binding could not be established (5).

Although the HZA provides an exciting investigational tool, its clinical usefulness has not been established. The requirements for human oocytes and the technical expertise involved in micromanipulation as well as expense involved limit the clinical usefulness of the HZA for the foreseeable future. Furthermore, the predictive value of the HZA would have to be developed for each site using it.

## LABORATORY PREPARATION

### Spermatazoa

Preparation of sperm for IVF can be based to some extent on sperm characteristics. The goal of preparations is to provide an adequate number of highly motile sperm and eliminate seminal contaminants and abnormal sperm. Many methods have been described for IVF.

The swim-up, the most commonly used method, involves sperm washing, then centrifugation to eliminate seminal plasma. The motile sperm can be retrieved by aspirating the media after 30–60 minutes of incubation. Variations to improve sperm recovery include fractionating the sample into several specimens to improve surface area, or by layering media directly over the unspun initial specimen. The motile sperm can then be resuspended in the proper concentration and volume for IVF (38). Recovery rates for this method are low, but there is a significant increase in percentage of motile cells and reduction in seminal contaminants (29).

Percoll centrifugation can be used in cases where there is a great amount of acellular debris or leukocytes in the semen sample (38). Percoll can be used as a continuous gradient but requires high-speed centrifugation. In a study by Berger, Marrs, and Moyer (4) comparing percoll discontinuous gradients with albumin gradient technique and swim-up techniques, the percoll gradient technique resulted in better motility (88% versus 81% versus 62%, respectively, for percoll, albumin, and swim-up), improved sperm recovery (59% versus 38% versus 18%), and enhanced performance in the hamster penetration assay.

In cases of severe oligospermia, a standard washing procedure is usually used to separate spermatazoa from the seminal plasma (8). This method calls for sample washing, centrifugation, and resuspension of the pellet. Although this technique allows better recovery, there is no selection for motility, and frequently debris or abnormal mucus is concentrated in the specimen. Generally, multiple tubes are used for the swim-up to maximize recovery.

## NEW TECHNIQUES

Investigators continue to look for techniques to enhance fertilization in couples with abnormal sperm function or concentration. Of these techniques, "microinjection" and "zona drilling" have received the greatest attention.

Microinjection involves placement of a capacitated spermatozoon in direct contact with the oolemma of the oocyte (19). A single sperm can be selected and inserted under the zona pellucida by microinjection. Fertilization and cleavage of human oocytes have been achieved with microinjection techniques (19). Although this technique provides hope for men with severely abnormal motility, concentration, or morphology, presently it is not adequately developed to be used clinically. Microinjection can be complicated by expulsion of injected sperm, oocyte damage, and perhaps parthenogenic activation of oocytes with resumption of oocyte meiosis due to oocyte injury (1, 19).

Furthermore, the procedure is technically complex and standard procedures have not yet been established. The use of microinjection also generates great numbers of questions and concerns. First, there is no known method to prospectively select an optimal or even a normal sperm with any degree of certainty. Although one might postulate that an abnormal sperm would not succeed in fertilizing the oocyte, no available data substantiates this conclusion. Many controversies that were discussed early in the development of IVF are likely to be reintroduced by this technique. These include concerns over genetic misadventures, medical treatment of humans without adequate assurance of safety, and financial expense. Microinjection remains an experimental technique for the treatment of male infertility at present.

Zona drilling uses micromanipulation to introduce a gap in the zona pellucida either mechanically or by localized application of a zona solvent from a microneedle. The procedure as described by Gordon and colleagues (14) initially requires cumulus dispersal. The zona is then "drilled" with one of several techniques—acid Tyrode's solution, pH 2–3, or alpha chymotrypsin loaded in a microneedle, which may be used to dissolve a local area in the zona. Alternately, zona intact oocytes may be incubated in chymotrypsin to soften the zona, and the zona can then be mechanically drilled using a microneedle. Fertilization followed by cleavage has been reported (4). Polyspermia is common and occurs in 50% of fertilized animal oocytes. There is also a concern that blastomeres may be lost through the hole in the zona and may result in developmental abnormalities. More data are required before this technique can be recommended for clinical therapy of infertile couples.

## CONCLUSION

IVF has given new hope to many couples unable to conceive due to abnormal semen parameters. Advances in sperm preparation and reports of new approaches provide further hope for the infertile couple. Before considering a couple for IVF, however, a thorough evaluation including history, physical exam, and appropriate testing as described earlier in the chapter must be performed. Donor insemination and adoption should be discussed with patients. Couples who are indeed candidates for IVF must be given realistic expectations of their chances of success. Referral to an IVF program established as a center capable of managing couples with severely abnormal semen parameters may be advised.

## REFERENCES

1. Acosta, A. A., et al. Assisted reproduction in the diagnosis and treatment of the male factor. *Obstet. Gynecol. Surv.* 44:1, 1989.
2. Ausmanas, M., et al. The zona-free hamster egg penetration assay as a prognostic indicator in a human in vitro fertilization program. *Fertil. Steril.* 43:433, 1985.
3. Awadalla, S. G., et al. In vitro fertilization and embryo transfer as a treatment for male factor infertility. *Fertil. Steril.* 47:807, 1987.
4. Berger, T., Marrs, R. P., and Moyer, D. L. Comparison of techniques for selection of motile spermatozoa. *Fertil. Steril.* 43:268, 1985.
5. Burkman, L. J., et al. The hemizona assay (HZA): Development of a diagnostic test for the binding of human spermatozoa to the human hemizona pellucida to predict fertilization potential. *Fertil. Steril.* 49:688, 1988.
6. Clarke, G. N., Elliott, P. J., and Sonada, C. Detection of sperm antibodies in semen using the immunobead test. A survey of 813 consecutive patients. *Am. J. Reprod. Immunol. Microbiol.* 7:118, 1985.
7. Cohen, J., et al. In vitro fertilization: A treatment for male infertility. *Fertil. Steril.* 43:422, 1985.
8. Corson, S. L., et al. The human-sperm-hamster egg penetration assay: Prognostic value. *Fertil. Steril.* 49:328, 1988.
9. Craft, I., et al. Sperm numbers and in-vitro fertilization. *Lancet* 2:1165, 1981.
10. Diamond, M. P., et al. Effect of the number of inseminating sperm and the follicular stimulation protocol on in vitro fertilization of human oocytes in male factor and non-male factor couples. *Fertil. Steril.* 44:499, 1985.
11. Dor, J., Rudak, E., and Aitken, R. J. Antisperm antibodies: Their effect on the process of fertilization studied in vitro. *Fertil. Steril.* 35:535, 1981.
12. Edwards, R. G., et al. Factors influencing the success of in vitro fertilization for alleviating human infertility. *J. In Vitro Fert. Embryo Transf.* 1:3, 1984.
13. Foreman, R., et al. The application of the zona-free hamster egg test for the prognosis of human in vitro fertilization. *J. In Vitro Fert. Embryo Transf.* 1:166, 1984.
14. Gordon, J. W., et al. Fertilization of human oocytes by sperm from infertile males after zona pellucida drilling. *Fertil. Steril.* 50:68, 1988.
15. Hargreave, T. B., and Elton, R. A. Treatment with intermittent high dose methylprednisolone or intermittent betamethasone for antisperm antibodies: Preliminary communication. *Fertil. Steril.* 38:586, 1982.
16. Hirsch, I., et al. In vitro fertilization in couples with male factor infertility. *Fertil. Steril.* 45:659, 1986.
17. Jones, W. R. Immunological factors in infertility. In R. J. Pepperell, B. Hudson, and C. Wood (eds.), *The Infertile Couple.* London: Churchill-Livingstone, 1986.
18. Junk, S. M., et al. The fertilization of human oocytes by spermatozoa from men with antispermatozoal antibodies in semen. *J. In Vitro Fert. Embryo Transf.* 3:350, 1986.
19. Laws-King, A., Trounson, A., Sathananthan, Kola, I. Fertilization of human oocytes by microinjection of a single spermatozoon under the zona pellucida. *Fertil. Steril.* 48:637, 1987.
20. Kruger, T. F., et al. Sperm morphologic features as a prognostic factor for in vitro fertilization. *Fertil. Steril.* 46:1118, 1986.
21. Kruger, T. F., et al. Predictive value of abnormal sperm morphology in in vitro fertilization. *Fertil. Steril.* 49:112, 1988.
22. Kuzan, F. B., et al. Human sperm penetration assay as an indicator of sperm function in human in vitro fertilization. *Fertil. Steril.* 48:282, 1987.
23. Leeton, J., et al. A controlled study between the use of gamete intrafallopian transfer (GIFT) and in vitro fertilization and embryo transfer in the management of idiopathic and male infertility. *Fertil. Steril.* 48:605, 1987.

24. Mahadevan, M. M., and Trounson, A. O. The influence of seminal characteristics on the success rate of human in vitro fertilization. *Fertil. Steril.* 42:400, 1984.
25. Mahadevan, M. M., Trounson, A. O., and Leeton, J. F. The relationship of tubal blockage, infertility of unknown cause, suspected male infertility, and endometriosis to success of in vitro fertilization and embryo transfer. *Fertil. Steril.* 40:755, 1983.
26. Mao, C., and Grimes, D. A. The sperm penetration assay: Can it discriminate between fertile and infertile men? *Am. J. Obstet. Gynecol.* 159:279, 1988.
27. Margalioth, E. J., et al. Zona-free hamster ovum penetration assay as a screening procedure for in vitro fertilization. *Fertil. Steril.* 40:386, 1983.
28. Margalioth, E. J., et al. Correlation between the zona free hamster egg sperm penetration assay and human in vitro fertilization. *Fertil. Steril.* 45:665, 1986.
29. McDowell, J. S., Veeck, L. L., and Jones, H. W., Jr. Analysis of human spermatozoa before and after processing for in vitro fertilization. *J. In Vitro Fert. Embryo Transf.* 2:23, 1985.
30. Rogers, B. J. The sperm penetration assay: Its usefulness reevaluated. *Fertil. Steril.* 43:821, 1985.
31. Rogers, B. J., et al. Variability in the human-hamster in vitro assay for fertility evaluation. *Fertil. Steril.* 39:204, 1983.
32. Rudak, E., et al. Assessment of the predictive ability of the zona-free hamster egg penetration test for the outcome of treatment by IVF-ET. *Int. J. Androl.* 6(Suppl.):131, 1986.
33. Van Uem, J. F. H. M., et al. Male factor evaluation in in vitro fertilization: Norfolk experience. *Fertil. Steril.* 44:375, 1985.
34. Wiley, L. M., et al. Detection of antisperm antibodies. Their localization to human antigens that are transferred to the surface of zona-free hamster oocytes during the sperm penetration assay. *Fertil. Steril.* 48:292, 1987.
35. Wolf, D. P., et al. Sperm concentration and the fertilization of human eggs in vitro. *Biol. Reprod.* 31:837, 1984.
36. Wolf, D. P., Sokoloski, J. E., and Quigley, M. M. Correlation of human in vitro fertilization with the hamster egg bioassay. *Fertil. Steril.* 40:53, 1983.
37. World Health Organization. *Laboratory Manual for the Examination of Human Semen and Semen-Cervical Mucus Interaction.* Cambridge: Cambridge University Press, 1987.
38. Yates, C. A. Male-factor infertility and in vitro fertilization. *J. In Vitro Fert. Embryo Transf.* 4:141, 1987.
39. Yovich, J. L., and Stanger, J. D. The limitations of in vitro fertilization from males with severe oligospermia and abnormal sperm morphology. *J. In Vitro Fert. Embryo Transf.* 1:172, 1984.

# Psychological Issues in IVF: Evaluation and Care

Peter J. Fagan and Yula Ponticas

A couple who is infertile suffers the frustration of the natural drive to procreate. Clinicians who work daily with infertile couples know well the emotional and interpersonal strain that this frustration causes some couples regardless of the specific etiology of the infertility. Involuntary childlessness is a condition in which the biologic and pscyhological factors interact, often producing significant emotional distress in the couple (8, 23). Clinical research suggests that the infertile couple is at risk for dysfunctional emotional distress (10), marital conflict (16), and sexual dysfunction (9).

Couples requesting in vitro fertilization (IVF) typically have been unsuccessful in their previous attempts at pregnancy. They are the "veterans" in the experience of infertility. Most have spent years undergoing medical examinations and evaluations; having intercourse on a schedule meant to maximize probability of conception; and responding to the ever-present social question, "When are you going to have a family?". Nearly 50% of the women and 15% of the men in a study of 200 consecutive IVF couples reported that infertility was the most upsetting experience in their lives (10).

Yet when couples apply for IVF they understandably attempt to present themselves in the most favorable light: desiring a child; having a stable marriage (if marriage is a requirement of the program); and being psychologically untroubled. For both personal and professional reasons, the IVF staff members want the applicants to be successful in the pursuit of biologic parenthood. The "best face forward" presentation on the part of the applicants and favorable staff predisposition can result in both applicants and clinicians being unaware of the degree of negative affect, e.g., depression or anxiety, that the couple may be experiencing as IVF is entered on (20). The emotional issues of IVF may be subtle clinically but important to the applicant couple.

This chapter suggests ways in which the subtle emotional and psychological needs of participants in IVF might be cared for by the IVF clinicians. We begin with a description of what the IVF participants experience as they go through the protocol and offer a model of psychological intervention. Then the psychological evaluation of IVF participants is described. In the final section, a word is offered to the IVF staff on an often neglected corollary of IVF: staff burnout.

## EMOTIONAL AND PSYCHOLOGICAL ISSUES DURING IVF

*IVF participant: "This opportunity, this notion unavailable just a few years ago has a way of calling you, rekindling hope when otherwise there would be none"(14).*

Although much has been written concerning the psychological characteristics of IVF candidates (10, 13, 22), little attention has focused on the emotional and psychological stress experienced by IVF participants as they proceed (or in some cases fail to proceed) through the IVF protocol. The components of the IVF procedure including induction of ovulation, oocyte retrieval, fertilization, and transfer provide the setting events for a variety of psychological reactions. Leiblum, Kemmann, and Lane (18) have offered a six-stage model of characteristic emotional, psychological, and physical reactions of IVF participants at each phase of the procedure. This model is based on psychometric data. Our clinical observations provide the framework for the present discussion of the psychological reactions that participants may experience during the IVF protocol.

## Acceptance into the Program

For many couples, acceptance into an IVF program is a point reached after several years of struggle with infertility treatment and the accompanying emotional and psychological stressors (21, 26). IVF represents the last option for some couples to become biologic parents. With this finality may be paired an urgency for the procedure to be successful, as well as the anxieties associated with realities such as waiting lists for and financial burdens of IVF programs (12). The reproductive technology of IVF may assume larger-than-life proportions as the couple's optimism for success far exceeds the statistical probabilities. Participants confide, "We know the numerical odds, but we are incredibly optimistic—each of us privately believes we are one of the chosen." Although a healthy degree of odds-beating optimism is perhaps necessary for IVF couples, expectations that admit no doubt lay the groundwork for future depressive reactions.

## Induction

Once the induction begins, daily administrations of menotropins (by clinician or husband), monitoring of serum estrogen levels, and frequent sonography represent the most disruptive elements of the IVF protocol in terms of time. Some participants have to travel great distances for the induction process, at times with the woman staying alone in a hotel close to the center when distance precludes the daily journey.

The frequency of visits to the IVF center during the induction process can interfere with family and job responsibilities, perhaps exacerbating the physical (fatigue, headaches, fluid retention, sore injection site) and emotional (labile mood, irritability) side effects of the menotropins. There is constant concern that the estrogen levels may not be adequately high, or conversely, that ovulation might occur too soon. Participants may find themselves comparing blood levels, sonography results, and physical exam findings with each other.

Induction failure due to inadequate estrogen levels or ovulation prior to scheduled retrieval of oocytes results in termination of the couple's participation in the IVF protocol. In many centers, this can mean a long waiting period before the next scheduled IVF cycle. This can result in anger and frustration, for participants may not expect termination this early in the process. The anger is often directed toward the clinicians for not tailoring the menotropin regimen to the woman's specific physiology, or for making errors in timing of ovulation with respect to scheduling of retrieval.

## Retrieval and Fertilization

The participants who proceed to the retrieval and fertilization phase of IVF often experience procedurally related stress (12). The retrieval can be more stressful than laparoscopies for infertility because of the burden the woman feels to produce the oocytes. Participants often worry about the maturity of the ova, or if all will be aspirated. These concerns can also be expressed indirectly through fear of the surgery/anesthesia, or anger may be projected on the clinician responsible for the retrieval should it be unsuccessful.

Fertilization requires that the man produce a semen sample on demand, and some men find this difficult to do. The assignment to produce a semen sample frequently reminds the man of providing a urine sample. Feelings of depreciation of his role on one hand and command performance on the other may result in resentment toward the physicians or performance anxiety.

When fertilization occurs, there can be anxiety and fear about proper cellular subdivision and growth. One participant, while awaiting results of the fertilization procedure articulated this point by saying, "I felt peculiar pangs of protectiveness that come with being a parent, even to offspring no bigger than a pencil point" (14). This reflects the profound emotional investment that participants may have in the outcome even prior to implantation. If the oocytes do not fertilize, the couple may question the integrity of their respective gamete contributions, their sense of inadequacy permeating to the cellular level. In the couple who has happily passed the retrieval hurdle, fertilization failure may more acutely bring to fore these feelings of anger, inadequacy, and loss.

## Transfer

After transfer, the woman must lie essentially immobile for 4–6 hours. One woman aptly summarized the immediate post-transfer experience: "It's awful. Worse was the feeling that my body was such an imperfect vessel, not nearly as safe and secure as the lab. I was afraid to get up after the six hours. What if the eggs spilled out?" (14). Some participants painfully acknowledge the tenuous nature of the post-transfer period. Others allow themselves to believe in the real possibility of biologic pregnancy, to the point where women report physical symptoms of pregnancy, such as breast tenderness and nausea (18).

## Failure

Negative pregnancy test, or more likely onset of the menses, is met with shock, as in the following experience of one of our participants: "Like others, I kept telling myself it couldn't happen to me. But it did, right on the tenth day. It hit me like a sharp sudden blow. I was stunned" (14). A period of intense denial of failure magnifies the anger, sadness, and great sense of emptiness that follows failure after a complete cycle of IVF participation. Amidst this sorrow, the question of "What next?" plagues many participants.

## Repeating IVF

The decision to repeat IVF, particularly after the first failure, is one that couples readily make, despite the emotional and psychological turmoil participation in the protocol can create. Many couples report that it is easier in subsequent attempts because the routine is a known one, physical settings and locations are familiar, and perhaps modifications in an individual procedure based on outcome of the initial trial give the participants a greater sense of control (e.g., specific dose of menotropins, use of pituitary suppressants). Couples may begin to realize that they, in fact, comprise the statistics that they believed they could overcome in their initial optimism. With repeated IVF attempts, we have seen at times a detachment of emotion to the procedure, with an almost mechanistic attitude toward achieving a biologic pregnancy. Other participants are progressively drained with successive attempts, and as one veteran participant phrased it, "The temptation is strong to blot out the whole subject like a bad dream" (14).

## Terminating IVF Attempts

Cessation of IVF attempts by a couple suggests that they have acknowledged that biologic pregnancy for them may not be an option given current technology. This acknowledgment by the couple comes after a period of grieving (21) not only for the child they may never produce, but for the biologic capacity to reproduce. The desire for a biologic child may never disappear; however it may be placed in a perspective that allows the couple, particularly the woman, to actively invest her energy in other generative endeavors. As one participant concluded, "For me, and I can only speak for myself on something so profoundly personal, it is more reasonable and more important to get on with other things" (19).

Some women who are infertile may put their life "on hold" until they achieve some satisfaction that they have tried everything available in reproductive technology to achieve biologic pregnancy. In a follow-up study of women who had completed one or more unsuccessful trials of IVF, Leiblum and colleagues (7) found that one-third of their sample had applied for adoption within 8 months of the decision to end IVF attempts, and over half felt that they had resolved the "crisis" of their infertility; however, 93% of these women stated that they would attempt any new reproductive technology that may give them the hope of achieving biologic pregnancy. This pervasive sentiment representing the drive to reproduce is captured very pointedly by one woman's perspective on IVF failure: "Even after all we've been through, it's not easy to turn down the chance for a miracle" (14).

Occasionally the couple's emotional struggle through the IVF process, particularly when there is failure, forces them to deal with buried conflicts and old wounds associated with past reproductive trauma or crises such as abortion, rape, stillbirths, miscarriage, infant death, molestation/abuse. One woman poignantly said, "IVF forced me to pull down my suitcase of old pain and open it. Now I have to unpack it, one piece at a time."

The IVF procedure will be experienced differently by each participant, with the emotional and psychological issues surfacing at differing points in the process based on individual history and vulnerabilities. The next section discusses ways in which IVF clinicians can assess and address these issues.

## PSYCHOLOGICAL INTERVENTION

Every interaction between an IVF clinician and patient is a psychological intervention. Phone conversations with the appointments secretary, correspondence with patients, the varied phone calls in times of distress, as well as the initial history aimed at understanding how the participants have coped with infertility are all psychological interventions. It is a matter of whether the communication between clinician and participant is helpful and therapeutic or not.

Annon and Robinson (2) have developed a model of interaction that has proved helpful in facilitating communication between clinicians and patient about sexual matters referred to as *PLISSIT,* an acronym for *P*ermission, *L*imited *I*nformation, *S*pecific *S*uggestions, and *I*ntensive *T*herapy.

First of all, the clinician gives the IVF participants *permission* to talk about the emotional issues that infertility has raised and IVF is raising in them. This *permission* is conveyed not only by direct questions, e.g., "How has all this been for you emotionally?", but also by a multitude of behaviors by which the clinician signals that he or she is ready and willing to listen to the emotional concerns that the patient may have. An unhurried examination, a follow-up question to what the patient says, and a description of the ways in which the IVF program offers psychological support to the patients and spouses are some of the ways in which permission is given to IVF participants to speak about their feelings and concerns to the IVF clinicians. The message is, "We want to hear how you are doing emotionally." Unfortunately, in the harried press of many clinical settings, this message is not given.

*Limited information* is a willingness in the clinician to convey to the participants information about the psychological reactions and issues that IVF may raise. It is limited only by the need and the ability of the participants intellectually and emotionally to understand the information. Examples of the psychological reactions have been discussed previously and described aptly by Leiblum and colleagues (18). Limited information has nothing to do with compromising the informed consent process; it has everything to do with allowing the participants to be aware of the reactions they may have (e.g., fatigue and fluid retention reaction to menotropin administration) as well as the decisions they may have to face (e.g., another IVF, adoption). Discussing and imagining an upcoming and emotionally charged event, especially when it involves medical or surgical procedures, may increase the anticipatory anxiety but seem to reduce negative effects during and subsequent to the event (1).

**Table 3-1. Psychosocial issues that may require attention by an IVF couple**

Cultural demand for parenthood
Pressure from parents to have grandchildren
Motivational discrepancy between spouses for having an IVF child
Sense of inadequacy in gender and sex roles
Sexual dysfunction secondary to infertility/IVF
Deferred career goals
Painful memories of incest, rape, abortion, sterilization
Religious/ethical concerns about IVF
Decision to accept childlessness or adoption

The sensitive clinician is able to give *specific suggestions* to participants on how they might cope with the stress connected with the IVF procedures. This is not a cookbook or "do's and don'ts" (though many suggestions will seem universal), rather recommendations reflective of this particular woman and her partner's situation. For example, who should be told that the couple is involved in an IVF protocol? Parents? Friends? Children of participants (potential siblings)?

Couples have varying needs for both privacy and support of others. An exploration of the quality of relationships the couple have with their own parents and friends will assist them to decide whether or not sharing the information with particular others will be helpful or not. If there is a great amount of pressure for grandchildren from parents, especially maternal parents, it is probably better to err on the side of postponing sharing the steps of the IVF protocol until a definite result is achieved (24).

Regarding existing children of the IVF couple, one must take into consideration whether or not they live in the home (stepchildren may be with the spouse of the previous marriage) and their age. If they are in the home of the IVF couple and of sufficient age to understand that "Mommy and Daddy are trying to have another baby with the help of the doctors," we suggest sharing this information. This gives them a way to understand the sacrifices that they are required to make during the IVF protocol (Mother's early morning and after-school trips to the doctors) as well as the "room" they will have to make psychologically and physically in the event of a birth.

These are but two areas in which specific suggestions can be helpfully given to the IVF participants. Of course, many other psychosocial areas require attention by a couple (Table 3-1). The clinician who listens closely to and learns from the successes and failures of previous patients, who is willing to get involved in the emotional concerns of his or her patient, can provide many helpful suggestions to IVF participants who are open to them.

A support group within the IVF program helps the participants to share their emotional reactions with true peers. Many of the specific suggestions about how to cope with the stress of IVF are shared very effectively, especially by those who have previously completed IVF. The same group dynamics as present in any group will be in an IVF support group. For example, issues of competition may surface, e.g., lab results, how many ova were retrieved, and so forth. These issues should be identified as reflecting competitiveness among group members and perhaps connected to other concerns about competition (especially with mothers and their own mothers) that group members may be experiencing. In general, we suggest that a person trained in group dynamics be the identified leader of an IVF support group and that the group be limited to eight members.

*Intensive therapy* for psychological conditions or psychosocial adaptation may be required by some participants in an IVF program as in any medicosurgical population. This can be provided in a structured manner either within the IVF program or by a referral to a mental health professional. In the latter case, the mental health professional should be familiar with both the psychosocial issues of infertility and the IVF protocol.

Increasing numbers of obstetrics and gynecology departments have full-time mental health professionals. The American Society of Psychosomatic Obstetrics and Gynecology (membership chair: Dennis H. Smith, M.D., 2105 Adelbert, Cleveland, OH 44106) is an association whose membership is drawn largely from clinicians who are interested in the psychological issues of obstetrics/gynecology patients. An IVF program is well served by having a mental health professional available for the treatment and management of individuals or couples who require more intensive therapy of a psychological nature. Frequently such a professional can help the staff to understand the patient better (e.g., "As an obsessive person, her anxiety will be expressed in a multitude of questions. . . . Be prepared."). He or she also serves as an identified "lightning rod" for the patient to process negative affect that otherwise might be directed toward the medical staff at inappropriate times.

The question of who should be referred to a mental health professional (either within the IVF program or in liaison with it) for more intensive therapy is a sensitive clinical decision and intervention. Hopefully the referral will be made before the patient's mental status deteriorates or patient-staff relations become so strained that it appears that the patient is being "sent to the shrink" as a form of punishment. To prevent this, all parties should be given a thorough psychosocial history, including past psychiatric history, before being accepted into the IVF program. If there is any indication of past psychiatric history, including alcohol or substance abuse; if the patient seems difficult to communicate with; or if, on mental status examination (15), there are neuronegative indications of affective illness (e.g., poor sleep and appetite, diurnal variation of energy and mood, poor memory and concentration), then a consultation from a psychiatrist or a psychologist should be obtained before accepting the person into the IVF program.

The IVF clinician should explain the reasons for the referral as directly as possible to the applicant. Often a clinician will experience awkwardness in making a psychiatric referral. This should diminish with the establishment of direct communication between professionals and, of course, competent and caring service rendered by the mental health professional.

## PSYCHOLOGICAL EVALUATION OF IVF PARTICIPANTS

Some IVF programs may choose to have a formal psychological evaluation as a routine step in the initial process of accepting an applicant into the IVF program. Either on referral for a specific patient or as part of the protocol, a psychological evaluation provides in a structured format the means of assessing the psychosocial strengths and limitations of the candidates. Properly interpreted and conveyed to applicants and IVF staff, the information gathered can assist participants and clinicians in their IVF collaboration. The evaluation can also identify those conditions requiring attention prior to participating in an IVF program, e.g., major depression and acute alcoholism.

The "referring question" of the IVF physician to the one performing the psychological evaluation is, "How will this applicant respond to a successful IVF or an unsuccessful IVF?". At some point in the interview, the applicants should be given the opportunity to explore both of these possibilities. By drawing on past events in their lives, the applicants should be assisted to expand on both outcomes. If she or they are unable to imagine an unsuccessful IVF, then these expectations should be labeled as unrealistic and described as such to applicants and staff. If other negative conditions coexist, e.g., history of major depression following previous miscarriages, these unrealistic expectations suggest deferring acceptance of the candidate into the IVF program until more realism is achieved.

The evaluation format that we employ has the following structure: (1) an interview with the couple together (15–20 minutes); (2) interview of each separately (1 hour); and (3) meeting with the couple together to give them impressions of the evaluation (15–20 minutes). This is only one of many formats that an evaluation may take. We find that this structure provides an opportunity to gain some understanding of both the interpersonal dynamics of the couple as well as the individual, intrapsychic dynamics of each partner.

The interview with the couple together is the initial contact between evaluator and a typically apprehensive and perhaps somewhat resentful ("Why do we have to go to a 'shrink' to have a baby?") couple. They should be told at the beginning of the interview that the purpose of the interview is to gain an appreciation of their psychological strengths and limitations as they might pertain to IVF; the information they reveal can be conveyed to the IVF physician; at the conclusion of the evaluation they will be told the evaluator's impressions and what his or her recommendation to the IVF physician will be; and finally, that the evaluator is available to them for psychological assistance throughout and following the IVF should they need it.

The interview with the couple together seeks to evaluate how they relate to each other, especially around the issue of infertility (4). An initial lead from the evaluator might be, "The two of you have been through a lot dealing with the infertility. I would be interested in hearing how it has been for you." Who does the talking? Is "blame" ascribed to one? How has the relationship been affected? Any loss of sexual interest in each other? How would either a successful or an unsuccessful IVF be handled? Does one want a child more than the other? Are there children in this marriage or through a previous marriage? What are the feelings each has as this IVF is attempted? Is there ambivalence? (If no, denial may be present.) Questions such as these generally provide information as well as engage the couple in the evaluation. At the conclusion of the initial interview, the couple typically feels that they are being listened to and that the sometimes previously ignored psychosocial stressors of infertility are being appreciated.

The individual interview consists of a full psychosocial history and mental status examination (15). Table 3-2 describes the psychosocial history components adapted from the psychiatric history outline used at Johns Hopkins Hospital. The mental status examination seeks to identify in a cross-sectional interview any symptoms of psychiatric disorder, especially affective illness, anxiety disorders, and formal thought disorders. At the conclusion of the individual interview, the evaluator should have impressions of (1) the general personality traits of the applicant; (2) history of any psychiatric illness in applicant or family; (3) presence of psychiatric disorder in applicant; (4) ego strength; (5) any motivational conflicts about IVF; and (6) available social supports as the individual begins the IVF protocol.

The final stage of the evaluation is sharing impressions of the evaluation with the couple. We suggest the "bottom line" be given first lest ignorance of it serve as a distractor to the participants. The three possible bottom line recommendations to the IVF physician are (1) to proceed with IVF with no psychiatric contraindications; (2) to proceed with IVF while concurrently addressing a specific condition, e.g., anxiety disorder, sexual dysfunction; (3) to defer IVF until a specific condition is corrected, e.g., acute alcoholism or major depression in the woman. The recommendation should be told to the couple and, if either of the latter two is given, a full exploration and possible suggestions/referrals should be made to the couple. This will obviously take more than the 15–20 minutes assigned to this part of the evaluation; however time spent here is vital for compliance with the recommendations to address a specified condition (which they may not have been aware of prior to the evaluation).

**Table 3-2. Outline of the psychosocial history employed in the interviewing of IVF applicants**

I. Family history
    Father, mother, siblings, extended family: age, health, education, occupation, personality, relationship with patient, alcoholism, psychiatric problems, diseases, neurologic and psychiatric problems
    Social position and family system
II. Personal history
    Gestational and perinatal events
    Timing of developmental milestones
    Unusual childhood illnesses (seizures, trauma, infection)
    Abnormal childhood behaviors (enuresis, stuttering, phobia)
    School history (academic performance, group activities, relationships with teachers and peers)
    Occupational history (terminations, job satisfaction)
    Living situations since leaving family of origin
    Menstrual and reproductive history
    Sexual development and behaviors
    Marital history(ies); health and status of children
    Habits (smoking, psychoactive substances)
    Religious affiliation and interest
    Medical history (presuming IVF physicians have complete hx)
    Psychiatric history
III. Infertility and IVF
    Previous reactions to infertility and treatment
    Expectations about present IVF attempt
    How will success/failure of IVF be handled?
    Final question: "Is there anything you would add to help me understand you better as you apply for IVF?"

When there are no psychiatric contraindications, time can be spent sharing with the couple specific impressions of them as a couple about to attempt IVF. Beginning with strengths, especially the strength of their marital union, is always a welcome confirmation. One can address then some of the limitations observed, e.g., not enough leisure and time together; a family history of depression that may be genetically linked; an incipient abuse of psychoactive substances, especially alcohol and cannabis.

The final word to the couple should be the restatement of the evaluator's availability to them should they require assistance during or subsequent to the IVF. Our experience has been that although most couples/individuals do not seek psychological assistance, approximately 5% have made requests for therapy or referrals following the IVF program.

## PSYCHOMETRIC EVALUATION OF IVF PARTICIPANTS

The use of standardized inventories to assess psychological and psychosocial conditions can greatly assist the IVF clinician in identifying participants who might have emotional difficulties during or subsequent to the IVF protocol. They should be employed in conjunction with the clinical interview and not as a replacement of it (3). We employ the following inventories to assist in the general psychological evaluation of participants: the NEO Personality Inventory (NEO-PI) (5); the Brief Symptom Inventory (BSI) (7); and the Michigan Alcohol Screening Test (MAST) (25).

NEO-PI (5) is a 181-item questionnaire developed through rational and factor analytic methods to operationalize normal personality traits in five broad dimensions: neuroticism, extraversion, openness to experience, agreeableness, and conscientiousness. Each of the first three domains encompasses a number of more specific traits. The NEO-PI scales have been related to measure normal personality traits, psychological well-being, and coping styles in normal populations. This makes the NEO-PI appropriate and helpful for the IVF population in keeping with the methodologic concerns raised by researchers (20) about the use of psychometric inventories with IVF applicants.

The BSI is a 53-item psychological self-report symptom scale developed from its longer parent instrument, the SCL-90-R (6). It is designed to assess the psychological symptom status of psychiatric and medical patients as well as individuals who are not patients. As a group, IVF women and their spouses scored within the nonclinical range (9). For this reason, we consider any individual scale score on the BSI above a total score of 60 (one standard deviation from the mean) to be worthy of clinical attention.

The MAST is a 25-item screening instrument to identify those with past or present patterns of alcohol abuse. Mindful of the unfortunate prevalence of alcohol abuse in the general population and of the effects of alcohol abuse on fetal development, we have found it to be a helpful instrument both for beginning discussion about drinking patterns with the IVF participants and for quantifying a clinical impression of alcohol abuse or dependence.

The NEO-PI, BSI, and MAST can be completed by the IVF participants in approximately 45 minutes. The NEO-PI can be computer scored with a textual commentary available through Psychological Assessment Resources, P.O. Box 998, Odessa, FL 33549.

## STAFF BURNOUT

During an IVF protocol, participants work closely with clinicians, at some points having daily contact. The stress in the IVF cycle does not reside solely in the participants. Clinicians involved in this intensely personal technology where failure far exceeds success and where scheduling and patients can be demanding have the potential to experience "burnout."

Professional burnout is characterized by loss of interest and motivation in the work, irritability, fatigue, and somatic complaints. Individuals experiencing burnout can become inflexible with regard to procedures and rules and lose their capacity to generate alternative solutions to problems. Goal driven, overdedicated personnel tend to be the most susceptible to burnout (11).

Clinicians involved in IVF are certainly not immune to these effects and are probably at a high risk for burnout given that they tend to be dedicated individuals motivated toward helping participants through the procedures. IVF clinicians often bear the brunt of participant anger, frustration, and hopelessness. Burnout can be avoided or caught early in its development by providing a forum such as a clinician group where the relevant issues can be processed together. Understanding one's limits as a clinician with respect to supporting participants through this difficult process, and knowing when to make a tactful referral to another professional (e.g., psychologist, psychiatrist) would help circumvent the complex and sensitive roles IVF clinicians assume.

## SUMMARY

IVF is a reproductive technology that provides many infertile couples with the possibility of biologic parenthood. Applicants to IVF programs typically have had years of the stress of infertility. They can be presumed to have psychiatric disorders equal to the prevalence found in the general population. As IVF participants, they will experience yet greater stress. Psychological intervention occurs throughout the program in every interaction between IVF staff and participants. Some special interventions are possible from IVF clinicians as well as formal psychological evaluation conducted by a psychiatrist or psychologist.

Finally, in the work of IVF, the staff must allow for special stress on its members and provide structural supports to avoid burnout.

## REFERENCES

1. Anderson, K. O., and Masur, F. T. Psychological preparation for invasive mental and dental procedures. *J. Behav. Med.* 6:1, 1985.
2. Annon, J. S., and Robinson, C. K. The use of vicarious learning in the treatment of sexual concerns. In J. LoPiccolo and L. LoPiccolo (eds.), *Handbook of Sex Therapy.* New York: Plenum, 1978,
3. Astor, J., and Pawson, M. The value of psychometric testing in the investigation of infertility. *J. Psychosom. Obstet. Gynecol.* 5:107, 1987.
4. Battaglia, A. R., Graziano, M. R., and Scafidi Fonti, M. G. Experimental research into the changes in the way sexuality is experienced by the infertile woman. *Acta Eur. Fertil.* 14:67, 1983.
5. Costa, P. T., Jr., and McCrae, R. R. *The NEO Personality Inventory Manual.* Odessa, FL: Psychological Resources, 1985.
6. Derogatis, L. R. The SCL-90 Manual I: Scoring, administration and procedures for the SCL-90. *Clin. Psycho.* Baltimore, 1977.
7. Derogatis, L. R., and Melisaratos, N. The Brief Symptom Inventory: An introductory report. *Psychol. Med.* 13:595, 1983.
8. Edelmann, R. J., and Connolly, K. J. Psychological aspects of infertility. *Br. J. Med. Psychol.* 59:209, 1986.
9. Fagan, P. J., et al. Sexual functioning and psychologic evaluation of in vitro fertilization couples. *Fertil. Steril.* 43:48, 1986.
10. Freeman, E. W., et al. Psychological evaluation and support in a program of in vitro fertilization and embryo transfer. *Fertil. Steril.* 43:48, 1985.
11. Freudenberger, H. J. *Burnout.* New York: Doubleday, 1980.
12. Greenfeld, D., et al. The role of the social worker in the in-vitro fertilization program. *Soc. Work Health Care* 10:71, 1984.
13. Hearn, M. T., et al. Psychological characteristics of in vitro fertilization participants. *Am. J. Obstet. Gynecol.* 156:269, 1987.
14. Hosler, K. Chance for a miracle. *Baltimore Sun Magazine,* 6 Jan. 1985, p. 8.
15. Kaplan, H. I., and Sadock, B. J. *Modern Synopsis of Comprehensive Psychiatry* (Vol. 4). Baltimore: Williams & Wilkins, 1985.
16. Lalos, A., et al. The psychosocial impact of infertility two years after completed surgical treatment. *Acta Obstet. Gynecol. Scand.* 64:599, 1985.
17. Leiblum, S. R., et al. Unsuccessful in vitro fertilization: A follow-up study. *J. In Vitro Fert. Embryo Transf.* 4:46, 1987.
18. Leiblum, S. R., Kemmann, E., and Lane, M. K. The psychological concomitants of in vitro fertilization. *J. Psychosom. Obstet. Gynecol.* 6:165, 1987.
19. Magida, L. Of reason and reproduction. *The Washington Post,* 29 May 1985, p. 14.
20. Mazure, C. M., De L'Aune, W., and DeCherney, A. H. Two methodological issues in the psychological study of in vitro fertilization/embryo transfer participants. *J. Psychosom. Obstet. Gynecol.* 9:17, 1988.
21. Menning, B. E. The emotional needs of infertile couples. *Fertil. Steril.* 34:313, 1980.
22. Morse, C. A., and Dennerstein, L. Infertile couples entering an in vitro fertilization program: A preliminary survey. *J. Psychosom. Obstet. Gynecol.* 4:207, 1985.
23. Morse, C. A., and Van Hall, E. V. Psychosocial aspects of infertility: A review of current concepts. *J. Psychosom. Obstet. Gynecol.* 6:157, 1987.
24. Sarrel, P. M., and DeCherney, A. H. Psychotherapeutic intervention for treatment of couples with secondary infertility. *Fertil. Steril.* 43:897, 1985.
25. Selzer, M. L. The Michigan Alcohol Screening Test: The quest for a new diagnostic instrument. *Am. J. Psychol.* 127:1653, 1971.
26. Shapiro, C. H. The impact of infertility on the marital relationship. *J. Contemp. Soc. Work* Sept., 387, 1982.

# The IVF-ET Team

# Personnel and the Organization of the IVF Team

Marian D. Damewood and Sharon G. Meng

The organization and implementation of an in vitro fertilization (IVF) team are time-consuming, often difficult undertakings. A working team not only requires the input and commitment of multiple individuals in both clinical and laboratory disciplines, but the cooperation and assistance of ancillary personnel in various departments with the hospital. Careful selection of personnel for an IVF team must take into account specific qualifications, of course, as well as the more important willingness to make a commitment to a program that often requires long hours, irregular schedules, and weekends. (1)

The outline of a working IVF team is shown in Figure 4-1. Of particular importance to an IVF team is the role of the nurse coordinator (3), which will be described in detail in the following paragraphs.

## APPLICATION TO THE IVF PROGRAM

The IVF nurse coordinator's responsibilities will be discussed in relation to the patient functions they accommodate. (2) The application process provides a good starting point. Information is disseminated to potential patients via direct phone calls, physician referrals, and response to written inquiries.

The coordinator participates in maintaining a waiting list of new patients wishing to enter the program. He or she then initiates a chart, makes a patient card for a card file, and acknowledges receipt of the application and entry to the waiting list using a form letter. Questions relative to the suitability of the patient for IVF are addressed to the medical director.

The coordinator also responds to inquiries by patients relative to their status on the waiting list. The card file is invaluable as a quick update source. A 3 × 5″ index card is completed on each patient, giving name, age, parity, diagnosis, primary care physician, date of application, and other pertinent data. Thereafter, conversations with the patient are noted on this card.

In addition, the coordinator meets with the medical director regarding patient selection. An acceptance letter and information packet is mailed to those patients who are selected to participate in the next cycle. Dates are specified by which the patient must confirm her participation and on which andrology screens and interviews may be scheduled. When a patient calls to accept, the coordinator schedules andrology and interview appointments and determines the expected date of the patient's menstrual period during the cycle.

## PRECYCLE

A certain amount of advance preparation is required prior to the start of the cycle. The coordinator must confirm the cycle dates with all ancillary services, including the sonography and phlebotomy departments, the special chemistry laboratory, the obstetrics/gynecology clinic, and the staffs of the operating room, recovery room, the antipartum inpatient unit, and nursing supervisors. The coordinator also works closely with the operating room nursing staff to ensure that all equipment required during oocyte retrievals is present and in working order.

IVF patient charts are set up in advance. Blank forms such as uterine sounding forms, ovulation induction flow sheets, consent forms, prescriptions, maps to the pharmacy, and financial forms are placed in the chart prior to the couple interview.

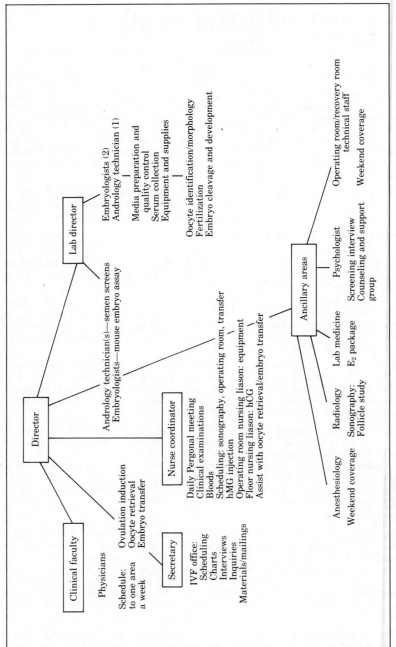

**Fig. 4-1. Outline of a working IVF team.**

## THE COUPLE INTERVIEW

After an interview with the medical director in which indications, medical history, risks, procedures, and consents are reviewed, the nurse coordinator meets with the patient to arrange the daily schedule. Arrangements for purchasing medications and receiving injections are formalized. If the patient is to give her own injections, a teaching session is scheduled for her and her husband on the day of her first Pergonal injection. If she will be receiving injections from an outside agency, the coordinator may need to make phone or written contact with this agency to provide instructions on reconstitution and injection sites. Patients are encouraged although not required to learn to self-inject, particularly for the progesterone supplementation post-transfer, stressing the increased autonomy and control this skill affords them.

Accommodations are discussed for out-of-town patients. These may include referral for appropriate housing locally and assistance in making arrangements such as confirming patient status, which will often result in a reduced rate.

## OVULATION INDUCTION

Patients are required to call the coordinator when their menstrual period begins, at which time they are instructed to begin injection of Lupron on day 20 of the cycle. An appointment is scheduled for a baseline ultrasound and estradiol level on the day prior to the first injection of gonadotropins. Appointments for monitoring the ovulation induction are also scheduled. Patients are reassured that although this is a complicated process, the coordinator will be in daily contact with them and each day will review the plan for the following day. Morning appointments are given at 7:30 A.M. in the gynecology and obstetrics clinic prior to normal office hours.

Each afternoon the secretary obtains the results of the morning's ultrasounds and estradiol assays. These are recorded by the coordinator on the ovulation flow sheets, which are then provided to each team member during the afternoon team meetings. If it is determined that patients are ready for surgery, the coordinator posts the surgery with the operating room and advises the andrology laboratory as well as the ultrasound technician. The coordinator then contacts the patient to arrange for her human chorionic gonadotropin injection at the appropriate time, reviews preoperative instructions, and makes an appointment for the final estradiol assay the following morning. Medical questions are referred to the physicians, thus allowing the coordinator to serve as a liaison between the physician and the patient.

## OOCYTE RETRIEVAL

The day prior to egg retrieval, the coordinator is responsible for reviewing preoperative instructions with the patient and scheduling the husband's appointment with the andrology lab to produce a specimen for oocyte insemination. He or she must be sure that operative consents are present in the chart and that the chart and consents are in the operating room. During the retrieval, the coordinator functions as part of the surgical team, assisting the physicians with oocyte aspiration.

## EMBRYO TRANSFER

On the day of the transfer it is the coordinator's responsibility to coordinate the time of the transfer with the embryologist, the physician, the operating room, and the patient and to reserve a room on the antipartum inpatient unit where the patient will subsequently rest. After the physician has reviewed the uterine sounding form in the patient's chart, the coordinator opens the necessary equipment (including a speculum, a tenaculum, a sterile container of Delbecco's solution, 3 × 4 sponges, a sponge stick, tuberculin syringes, and a tomcat catheter) and assists the physician with the transfer. Following the procedure, the patient is assisted onto a stretcher and is transferred to the antipartum room where she will rest for 4 hours.

In summary the role of the IVF nurse coordinator is to work closely with the medical director to facilitate the IVF process and to provide a vital link between the physicians, the patients, and all ancillary services interacting with the program.

## REFERENCES

1. Garner, C. H. Establishing and working in an IVF program. *Insights into Infertility,* June 2, 1985 (syllabus) Serono.
2. Pepperell, R. J., et al. The role of the SW and nursing practitioner in infertility care. In *The Infertile Couple.* New York: Churchill-Livingstone, 1987.
3. Peindl, C. The expanding nursing role in infertility. *Insights into Infertility,* June 2, 1985 (syllabus) Serono.

# IVF Office Procedure

Marian D. Damewood and Teresa M. Zemanski

The first contact a prospective patient for the in vitro fertilization (IVF) program has is the office secretary. The prospective patient calls the office inquiring about IVF. The secretary explains the general day-to-day workings of the program and then asks the prospective patient if she would like an application mailed to her. The secretary will then mail the IVF information packet and also inform the prospective patient that she must get copies of her medical records and send them to the IVF program along with the filled-out application (Fig. 5-1). On receiving the medical records and completed application, the information is then forwarded to the IVF nurse coordinator who will make a chart on the prospective patient and add her to the waiting list.

The nurse coordinator keeps a waiting list for the IVF program. When the dates are selected by the IVF program director for a cycle to start, the nurse coordinator and IVF director will meet and review the IVF patient charts to select the patients for that cycle. Then the selection list is given to the secretary who looks up the addresses on the computer and sends a letter stating that the patient has been selected for an IVF cycle. Detailed information packets stating step-by-step exactly what will be done during this IVF cycle are sent. The patient is informed that she must respond to the nurse coordinator by a certain date as to whether she would like to go through the program at this time. When the patient contacts the nurse coordinator, appointments are set up for the patient to sign the consent forms, review any questions, and for the husband's semen screen.

Once the cycle has started, the secretary will retrieve the ultrasound reports for daily follicular monitoring from the ultrasound department. He or she will then retrieve the estradiol blood results from the special chemistry lab and give these results to the nurse coordinator who will put these results on the ovulation induction form and give them to the secretary to photocopy for the ovulation induction meeting. During this meeting the IVF director and staff review the results and decide the amounts of medications to give each patient. The patients are contacted between 2:30 and 3:00 P.M. each day to get these results along with the amount of medication they should take for that day.

When the patients are unable to get in touch with the nurse coordinator during the day, they are advised to call the IVF office and leave a message for either the IVF director or IVF nurse coordinator. The secretary serves as back-up in scheduling the operating room surgery. The director will tell the secretary that the patient will be having her oocyte retrieval on a specified day. The secretary will then contact the operating room with the patient's name, history number, telephone number, and time of surgery. He or she will then contact the anesthesia department and IVF lab personnel to let them know of the surgery. The secretary is also responsible for coordinating and tabulating the pregnancy tests and results on each patient.

Johns Hopkins Hospital
In Vitro Fertilization Waiting List Application

Date _____          Gynecologist _____
                                        GYN Address  _____
                                        GYN Phone    _____


Last Name _____          Home Phone _____
Address _____


                    WIFE                                    HUSBAND


First Name _____          _____
Birth Date _____          _____
Height and Weight _____          _____
Allergies _____          _____
Occupation _____          _____
Work Phone _____          _____
Insurance _____          _____
Social Security No. _____          _____


Infertility

Diagnosis _____          _____
          _____          _____
          _____          _____

Previous surgeries and dates

          _____          _____
          _____          _____
Medications _____          _____
          _____          _____


Menstrual History
Average cycle length _____
Average day of ovulation _____
Number of previous pregnancies _____
Number of previous deliveries _____

Are you in a position to spend the necessary time and expense in Baltimore?
_____

Have you been a patient at the Johns Hopkins Infertility Clinic? _____
If so, date of last visit. _____

Comments: _____
_____
_____

**Fig. 5-1. Johns Hopkins Hospital In Vitro Fertilization Waiting List Application.**

# Appendix 5-1. Johns Hopkins Hospital IVF Protocol

The following schedule and instructions may answer some of your questions about your upcoming IVF cycle.

## IVF SCHEDULE

### Cycle Before IVF Attempt

Call Nurse Coordinator and let him or her know your period has started so the date of starting lupron may be arranged (day 20 of cycle prior to IVF attempt).

### Day 10 of Lupron

Arrive 7:30 A.M. for blood drawing and sonogram. You will have both an abdominal and vaginal sonogram.

### *Medications*

You will be given prescriptions at the time of your interview that must be filled prior to the start of your cycle. Daily injections will be given at the hospital or the satellite office, or you may arrange for a friend, relative, or other health care provider to give them. The Nurse Coordinator will be glad to lend you a videotape demonstrating injection technique. If you are receiving your injections at the hospital/satellite office, you must bring your medications with you. If you have made alternative arrangements, you must be accessible by phone between 2:30 and 3:30 P.M. daily. All medications must be taken at 4 P.M. Medication dosages are as follows:

| | |
|---|---|
| Lupron | 1 mg (0.2 cc) prior to your induction, 0.5 mg (0.1 cc) during your induction. Lupron is discontinued the day of human chorionic gonadotropin (hCG). |
| Pergonal | Two to four ampules as directed daily. |
| Metrodin | Two ampules on days 1 and 2 of induction. |
| hCG | 10,000 units as directed. |
| Progesterone | 25 mg (0.5 cc) twice daily post egg retrieval. |
| hCG | 5000 units 2 days after the embryo transfer. |

You will be receiving high doses of hormones. Side effects of these medications include headaches, mood swings, loss of appetite, abdominal fullness and tenderness, and muscle soreness at the injection site. The latter may be relieved by massage after the injection, local application of heat, and walking. *It is critical* that you use barrier contraception (condom, diaphragm) in the cycle in which you begin your Lupron injections.

| | | |
|---|---|---|
| 8–9–10 | A. | When tests indicate you are close to ovulation, stop taking Pergonal per instructions. You will still need to have your blood drawn daily until your retrieval. |
| | B. | Husband should ejaculate 2–3 days before egg retrieval as directed. Check with nurse coordinator for timing. |
| | C. | You will be notified when to take hCG and when your egg retrieval is scheduled. |
| 36 hours later | A. | Follow preoperative instructions. |
| | B. | Report to OR for ultrasound-directed oocyte retrieval 2 hours before your surgery is scheduled. Husband will go to lab to give semen specimen. Time will be arranged through nurse coordinator. |
| Following day | A. | Take first evening injection of progesterone. |
| | B. | You will be notified of probable time of transfer. |

Transfer day    A. Take first morning injection of progesterone.
                B. Report to Nelson 2 GYN/OR area at assigned time.
                C. Follow pre/post-transfer instructions.
                D. Take evening injection of progesterone. Continue with two
                   injections daily at established times.
                E. Try to rest as much as possible transfer day and next three
                   days. Normal activities may then be resumed, avoiding
                   vigorous exercise and heavy lifting. Do not resume sexual
                   relations until after pregnancy test.

Six days after first injection of hCG: injection of 5000 units of hCG. 14 days
later: Come to the hospital to have a pregnancy test drawn.

**Remember**

1. You will have a sonogram on day 10 of lupron. If this will be your first
   sonogram at Johns Hopkins, or if you have not had an abdominal sonogram
   within the last 6 months, *please* arrive at the hospital with a full bladder
   and do not empty your bladder until after this procedure is completed. For
   subsequent sonograms you will be examined using the vaginal transducer,
   which does not require a full bladder.
2. The daily blood test is *critical* to the success of the IVF process. Blood can
   only be drawn between 7:30 and 8:30 A.M. on Monday through Friday and
   9:30–10:00 A.M. on weekends *with no exceptions!*
3. Please refrain from intercourse after cycle day 4. Husbands should ejaculate
   2–4 days before egg retrieval so that the best possible specimen for fertilizing
   the eggs will be available. Discuss timing for ejaculation with Nurse Coordinator.
4. Please bring your hospital plate any time you come to the hospital.
5. Please purchase your medications *before* your cycle starts and store according
   to enclosed directions. Do not forget to bring medication with you when you
   come to the hospital for injections.
6. If you desire to receive your injections at home, you and the person giving
   the injections will need to be at the hospital on cycle day 1 at 4 P.M. for an
   instructional session. Make an appointment with the Nurse Coordinator.
7. Those receiving injections outside the hospital should be available by phone
   daily between 2:30 and 3:30 P.M. to be advised of dosages and test results.
   We may not be able to answer other questions during this hour but will be
   glad to call you back later or in the morning.
8. After egg retrieval, we will keep you informed on the progress of your eggs/
   embryos and the projected time for the transfer; however, as the eggs generally make little if any progress in the first day, please do not call until at
   least 24 hours have passed.
9. If you have medical complications/concerns, these should be addressed to the
   physicians. The Nurse Coordinator is available by phone for questions, problems, or just to talk.
10. We will try to keep you and your husband as well informed as possible
    throughout the IVF process. Each IVF participant is a unique and special
    person; therefore, the program is individualized to meet each woman's par-
    ticular needs. Because no two women respond in quite the same way, we
    encourage you not to compare results and not to be disheartened or overly
    optimistic by any disparities you may discover.
11. The medications will include Metrodin (pure follicle stimulating hormone)
    to start, followed by Pergonal (human menopausal gonadotropin). You may
    also be put on lupron. The IVF Director will decide on the doses of medication
    according to each individual patient's response.

## IVF AMBULATORY SURGICAL CENTER POSTOPERATIVE INSTRUCTIONS

Remember to take the antibiotic prescribed to you for 48 hours if you have a laparoscopy.

Transfer of oocytes will take place 48 hours post discharge from the outpatient department area. The IVF team will be notifying you 24 hours in advance. Progesterone injections will be taken morning and evening, 12 hours apart beginning with the evening injection on the day after surgery.

Please contact the IVF Coordinator with any questions.

When you go home after surgery is finished, take it easy for the rest of the day. Do not attempt to do anything that requires skill or coordination such as driving, working with a power tool, etc. Do not make important decisions for 24 hours.

Begin to drink clear liquids (Coke, iced tea, jello, etc.) as tolerated, and go on to a light meal if you feel like it.

Do not drink alcoholic beverages until 24 hours after anesthesia and the operative procedure.

A tired, washed-out feeling may last for 1 to 2 days if you have general anesthesia. It is due to both the anesthesia and the operative procedure. This is normal. You may have a sore throat for the first 24 hours after your procedure if you have had general anesthesia. This is harmless and will disappear. It can be relieved by using a standard nonprescription throat lozenge or gargle.

In addition, you may have some mild pain from your procedure. You may take extra-strength Tylenol for pain. Notify your physician about any increase in pain that is not controlled by the pain medication. Postoperatively, if any questions arise concerning your anesthetic, you may call the Anesthesiologist on-call.

There may be soreness, light bleeding, or oozing from the incision if you have a laparoscopy. This is due to the incision and the sutures used to close it. The soreness may last about 1 week. There is no cause for alarm. Simply change the dressing as instructed and keep the incision clean as instructed for 5–7 days. Your physician will have told you whether you may shower or tub bathe. Please call your physician if you notice any signs of infection, i.e., redness, pus, swelling.

With ultrasound retrieval, a feeling of abdominal fullness may persist for a few days. In addition, you may experience some mild abdominal cramping or spotting.

## IVF POST-TRANSFER INSTRUCTIONS

A slightly bloody discharge may be seen after the transfer procedure. This is a normal occurrence. Excessive discharge or bleeding, pain, or fever must be reported immediately to the Nurse Coordinator or one of the physicians.

For 3 days post-transfer, no strenuous activity is advised. Try to rest as much as possible. Any specific questions concerning activity can be addressed to the physicians. Injection of 5000 units of HCG will be given 2 days after embryo transfer.

Progesterone injections are to be taken twice daily 12 hours apart. You may set your own schedule for these injections. For convenience, we recommend that you or your husband learn to give these injections.

14 days post-transfer you will be required to return to the hospital for a blood pregnancy test. A date will be confirmed with you post-transfer.

Any questions concerning the above can be addressed to the IVF Nurse Coordinator.

## SEMEN COLLECTION FOR INTRAUTERINE INSEMINATION AND IVF

1. Abstain from ejaculation for 2 days if you have a normal count, 3–4 days prior to collection if your count is low.
2. Come to the Reproductive Endocrinology Laboratory.

3. The technician in the laboratory will provide a specimen container and answer any further questions at that time.
4. *Do not* use a condom for collection.
5. *Do not* use creams or lubricants during collection.
6. Please deliver the specimen to the laboratory as soon as it is collected. The specimen container should remain upright at all times, and care should be taken to ensure that the lid is tightly secured.
7. Please be sure that your name and your wife's name are clearly labeled on the container.
8. Please feel free to ask the laboratory personnel any questions about collection of the sample. They are all highly professional and may be able to help allay any concerns that you may have.
9. If you are unable to produce a specimen in the hospital environment, please talk to the Nurse Coordinator so that alternative arrangements may be made.

# Appendix 5-2. The Johns Hopkins Qualifications for Entry into IVF Program

1. Infertility resulting from removal of both fallopian tubes, persistent infertility despite surgical therapy for tubal disease or endometriosis, untreatable cervical factor, oligospermia, and unexplained infertility.
2. Weight must be appropriate for height.
3. Patients must complete the enclosed application and have pertinent medical records forwarded to this office.

## THE IVF PROGRAM

The program of in vitro fertilization has various names. It has also been referred to as "test-tube baby" program or extracorporeal fertilization. Its purpose is to achieve a pregnancy for those couples who cannot become pregnant and who have tried and failed with conventional methods of therapy.

For a pregnancy to result through IVF, four separate procedures must be successfully completed:

1. Hormonal stimulation to develop the eggs
2. Retrieval of eggs
3. Fertilization of egg with sperm
4. Transfer of the embryo into the mother's uterus

If just *one* step of the procedure fails, pregnancy cannot occur.

### Hormonal Stimulation of the Egg

Well-developed eggs are needed from the ovaries to proceed with in vitro fertilization. Egg development will be accomplished by administering fertility drugs at the beginning of a menstrual cycle. Egg development will be monitored by measuring the changes of hormones in the blood and performing pelvic sonograms and pelvic examinations.

### Egg Retrieval

When the egg is mature, it must be removed from the ovary. To do this, a transvaginal ultrasound-guided oocyte retrieval is performed under intravenous sedation, and the eggs are taken from the ovary using a suction apparatus. In some cases, the patient's anatomy may necessitate a laparoscopy for egg retrieval, which is a surgical procedure performed under general anesthesia.

### Fertilization of Egg and Sperm

After one or more eggs are obtained, they must be fertilized in the laboratory. A sperm specimen must be obtained from your husband. Fertilization takes place in the laboratory, in an incubator. Development will be allowed to proceed for about 48–72 hours. As in the normal situation, sometimes fertilization does not occur even when the egg and sperm meet, or in some instances, development begins but then stops. This happens in normal fertilization, but it is not known if it is more frequent in the laboratory. A fertilized egg is known as an *embryo*.

### Transfer of the Embryo into the Uterus

After a short period of development the early embryo or egg must be transferred into the uterus. This is done by a small transfer catheter and is a relatively simple procedure similar to a pelvic examination. The transfer process, however, is very inefficient. It is not known why many early developing embryos are transferred but fail to develop within the uterus.

### Implantation of the Embryo into the Uterus and Nurturing of the Embryo

In the normal process of fertilization, the early implantation of the embryo in the uterus is under the control of the corpus luteum, which is a small gland in the ovary at the site of the follicle where the egg had matured. In view of the fact that it is necessary to aspirate this follicle, it is unknown whether the normal development of the corpus luteum is hampered. It is considered advisable to supplement the function of the corpus luteum by the administration of progesterone daily by injection.

It is important that those who enter the program understand that the chance of success in any one fertilization is small. Normal fertile couples achieve pregnancy in the natural way after an *average* exposure of 3 months, with a range of one exposure up to several months or even years. It is unlikely that the IVF program will be able to improve on the biologic circumstances that make an average of three exposures necessary. The expectation of pregnancy in any one attempt in the IVF program will be less than the normal average.

### IF PREGNANCY OCCURS:

One of the questions often asked is, what is the expectation of an abnormal child? Unfortunately, under entirely normal circumstances, the birth of abnormal children occurs. A committee appointed by the Secretary of Health, Education and Welfare considered many aspects of IVF, including the question of whether an increased number of abnormal children would be born by the IVF process. The committee concluded that it would be unlikely that this would occur, but of course, no assurances can be given.

### TIME INVOLVED

An IVF attempt from hormone stimulation through pregnancy test lasts approximately 6 weeks. You will be seen daily at the hospital for at least 2 weeks including your egg retrieval and embryo transfer.

# Informed Consent for IVF Procedures

## Marian D. Damewood

For any surgical procedure, informed consent is of utmost importance in patient management and guidance. Although some patients may be aware of the specifics of the procedure being performed, the potential outcome and the possible complications that may be associated with the procedures must be reviewed in detail. As with most surgical procedures, obtaining informed consent involves a careful explanation of the procedure to the patient along with its inherent risks and benefits.

Unlike a single surgical procedure, in vitro fertilization (IVF) procedures involve a minimum of a four-step process. Initially induction of ovulation is performed with various types of fertility agents. This requires a separate consent for the administration of fertility drugs to induce ovulation along with the inherent risks of ovarian hyperstimulation or drug allergy. The second part of the IVF procedure is the oocyte retrieval, which can be performed either laparoscopically or by ultrasound guidance. The individual patient problem may dictate which retrieval technique is performed; however the patient should be familiar with both aspects of retrieval techniques, since in some cases an oocyte retrieval may not be able to be performed easily and a laparoscopy must be done.

The most complex aspect of informed consent for IVF involves the laboratory aspects. Although a separate consent form is not obtained for fertilization and embryo development, this procedure is explained in detail to the patient at the initial consultation and throughout the IVF procedure. A specific individual consent form may be obtained from the patient who has a request such as all embryos be transferred back to the uterus or a specific number of embryos for transfer back to the uterus. In addition, cryopreservation of embryos will require a separate consent form.

The embryo transfer, a simple gynecologic procedure, is included in the consent forms for surgical procedures associated with IVF. The consent forms used at the Johns Hopkins In Vitro Fertilization Program were prepared with the guidance of the legal office and In Vitro Fertilization Program Team (Fig. 6-1).

Authorization (or consent) for Administration
of Anesthesia and for Performance of Operations
or other Procedures

PATIENT_____DATE_____TIME_____ A.M. P.M.

I hereby give my consent and authorize Doctor_____

of The Johns Hopkins Hospital to perform the following operation or other procedure:

Ultrasound-directed vaginal retrieval

Diagnostic/operative laparoscopy, follicular puncture, lysis of adhesions,

fulguration of endometriosis

Identify and explain in non medical terms, use no abbreviations

I acknowledge that:

1. The nature and purpose of the operation or other procedure and anesthesia, the risks involved, alternatives, and the possibility of complications have been explained to me by Doctor_____ and all my questions, if any, have been answered to my satisfaction. I am aware that the practice of medicine and surgery is not an exact science, and I acknowledge that no guarantee has been made as to the results that may be obtained.

2. I consent to the performance of the above-named operation or other procedure and if, during the contemplated operation or other procedure, other conditions are discovered that, in the best judgment of the medical staff of The Johns Hopkins Hospital, require an extension of the original contemplated operation or other procedure or a different operation or other procedure, I authorize and request that the said operation or other procedure be performed.

3. I further consent to the administration of such anesthesia as may be considered necessary or advisable in the judgment of the medical staff of The Johns Hopkins Hospital.

4. Exceptions to surgery or anesthesia, if any, are:_____
(If "none", so state)

5. I consent to the disposal by authorities of The Johns Hopkins Hospital of any tissues or parts which it may be necessary to remove. I authorize The Johns Hopkins Hospital to retain, preserve, and use for scientific or teaching purposes any tissue or specimens taken from my body.

6. I consent to the admittance of observers, in accordance with ordinary practices of The Johns Hopkins Hospital, to the use of closed-circuit television, the taking of photographs (including motion pictures), and the preparation of drawings and similar illustrative graphic material, and I also consent to the use of such photographs and other materials for scientific purposes, provided my identity is not revealed by the pictures or by the descriptive text accompanying them.

7. The undersigned acknowledges receipt of a copy of the foregoing consent and authorization to an operation or other procedure.

_____                    _____
Witness's Signature                          Patient's Signature

_____          JHH ID NO. ☐ ☐  ☐ ☐  ☐ ☐
Signature of Physician Securing Consent

IF PATIENT IS UNABLE TO SIGN OR IS A MINOR, COMPLETE THE FOLLOWING:

Patient(is a minor_____ years of age) or is unable to sign because:

_____                    _____
Witness's Signature                          Closest Relative or Legal Guardian's Signature

JHH 15-144020

A

**Fig. 6-1. Preoperative consent forms for the Johns Hopkins IVF Program.**

02    STAMP PATIENT'S IDENTIFICATION OR PRINT CLEARLY
Nursing Unit Clinic                                    Date Initiated

03                        J.H.H. - History Number

**THE JOHNS HOPKINS HOSPITAL**

04
Patient's Name (Last, First, M.I.)

**INFORMED CONSENT SUPPLEMENT**

I.    INDICATIONS FOR THE OPERATION OR OTHER PROCEDURE ARE:
    Infertility

II.   MAJOR RISKS OF THE OPERATION OR OTHER PROCEDURE AND ANESTHESIA (including such items as failure to obtain the desired result, discomfort, injury, additional therapy and death):
    Bleeding requiring transfusion; infection requiring antibiotics; damage

    to bowel, blood vessel, or bladder requiring laparotomy; excessive bleeding

    from the ovary requiring laparotomy; anesthesia risk.

III.  Alternatives to the proposed operation or other procedure
    No surgery.

IV.   In instances where a discussion of the above is deemed unwise medical practice, there should be documented a statement to this effect below, stating the reason for this decision (This space may also be used for explanatory diagrams.)

_____
Witness's Signature

_____
Patient's Signature

_____
Signature of Physician Securing Consent

JHH ID NO.

The undersigned acknowledges receipt of a copy of the foregoing Informed Consent Supplement for an operation or other procedure this

_____ day of_____ 19_____

_____
Witness's Signature

_____
Patient, Closest Relative, or Legal Guardian's Signature

JHH 15-144040

B

# Appendix 6-1. Consent Forms

**Consent to the Use of Drugs to Induce Ovulation, and the Use of Ultrasound Techniques for Evaluation of Developing Follicles**

I understand that I will receive a daily intramuscular injection of a fertility drug to stimulate the development of many eggs. The length of treatment depends on my response to the medication as determined by blood and sonogram studies, but may range between 6 to 14 days. The eggs develop inside fluid-filled cysts called follicles. As the follicles grow, the ovary secretes increasing amounts of estrogen. Daily blood specimens will be taken from my vein for not less than 10 days to measure blood estrogen levels and possibly other hormones. At an appropriate time during the course of treatment, sonogram (ultrasound) studies will be performed to measure the size of the ovarian follicles. I understand that there are no known risks to me or my eggs with the use of ultrasound. My doctor will interpret these studies to determine how the eggs are developing.

The risks of repeated blood sampling include skin irritation and small bruises. The medication to be given is identical in chemical structure to the hormones produced by the body that normally stimulate ovulation. Stimulation of the ovaries from the hormone therapy may occasionally cause ovarian enlargement, abdominal pain, and fluid retention in the abdomen and lungs. When these types of fertility drugs were used many years ago, extreme over-stimulation was associated with rupture of the ovaries in a few patients, which resulted in removal of the ovaries. This occurred before the availability of ultrasound monitoring and has not been reported in the last twenty years. Because of the possibility of side effects, I understand the importance of remaining in close communication with my doctors during the course of my injections and for approximately 10 days following ovulation.

I understand that my participation may contribute to the general advancement of scientific knowledge that may benefit some individuals in the future. I understand that any information obtained by my use of the fertility drugs may be used in medical studies, however, my name will be kept confidential. I understand that my diagnostic studies will be supervised by one of the investigators and that the Program Director will oversee my care.

I am advised that if physical injury should result from participation in this program, the Johns Hopkins University and Hospital provide no insurance coverage, compensation plan, or free medical care plan to compensate me for such injuries.

I understand that photographs of my abdomen, or pelvic organs, may be taken. I understand that the purpose of these photographs is to teach other physicians. I understand that my confidentiality will be protected.

I, _____, hereby give permission to the physicians at The Johns Hopkins Hospital to direct an injection of pituitary gonadotropin daily as prescribed, and to obtain blood and sonogram studies as indicated.

It is, of course, understood that even after signing this consent form I may withdraw from the program without prejudicing my future therapy or clinical care.

Patient's Signature _____ Date _____

Witness' Signature _____ Date _____

I have explained the above to the subject on the date stated on this consent form.

Physician's Signature _____ Date _____

## IN VITRO FERTILIZATION CONSENT FORM

*In vitro fertilization* (IVF) or "test-tube baby" refers to the program where an egg (oocyte) is removed from the ovary, taken to the laboratory and mixed with sperm, to allow fertilization. Following fertilization, a very small embryo (two to eight cells) will form, and be transferred back into the womb where it will hopefully grow into a normal pregnancy. This program will be available to only those women who cannot conceive by any other means.

To perform IVF, hormones that are normally present in the body are injected into the woman on a daily basis during the early phase of the menstrual cycle to stimulate the development of eggs in the ovaries. The eggs grow inside fluid-filled cysts called follicles. Egg development will be monitored by drawing a small blood sample (one tube) daily and by using "ultrasound" (sonography) to measure the size of the ovarian follicles. At the correct time, a laparoscopy or ultrasound vaginal retrieval is performed under general or local anesthesia to remove the eggs from the ovaries. These eggs are then mixed with the husband's sperm to allow fertilization. When fertilization has occurred and a small embryo is formed, it is transferred into the womb using a very small tube.

Certain major and minor risks are associated with IVF. These are listed below.

### Major Risks

1. Overstimulation of ovaries from hormone therapy causing severe abdominal pain, fluid retention in the lungs, and under extreme circumstances, death. This problem has not yet occurred in women undergoing IVF.
2. Complications of the diagnostic laparoscopy are the same as those present whenever this procedure is performed. These include anesthesia complications; infection; bleeding; injury to bowel, bladder, uterus, blood vessels, or other pelvic organs.
3. Complications of transvaginal, ultrasound-guided egg retrieval include injury of any pelvic structures with the needles, including blood vessels, bowel, bladder, uterus, tubes, and ovaries. In very rare instances this could require surgical repair. There is also a small chance of infection.
4. Failure of the procedure. Despite all efforts, it might be impossible to grow an egg, remove it from the ovary, or fertilize it with sperm. Even if the egg is fertilized, it may not grow and become a normal pregnancy. The best results obtained to date indicate a successful pregnancy rate of only 15–20%.
5. Possibility of an "ectopic" pregnancy. If a pregnancy occurs, there is a small chance (less than 1%) that the pregnancy could form in the fallopian tube or abdomen. If this occurred, major surgery to remove the pregnancy would be necessary.
6. Possibility of birth defects. An increased risk of birth defects in IVF pregnancies has not been reported. The usual risk of a birth defect during a "normal" pregnancy is 3–5%. No guarantee can be given if a pregnancy results from IVF that a birth defect will not be discovered at birth or many years after.
7. Multiple births. Since more than one fertilized egg is usually transferred back into the womb, it is possible that a twin or triple pregnancy may occur.

### Minor Risks

1. Irritation, infection, or injury at the site of hormone injections.
2. Irritation or infection at the site used for diagnostic laparoscopy.
3. Irritation, infection, or allergic reaction following transfer of the embryo into the womb.

The IVF program is designed to allow pregnancy when it could not happen under any other conditions between husband and wife. Because of this, any alternative to IVF should be considered. For example, surgery to correct the fallopian tubes may be possible in hopes of achieving pregnancy prior to considering IVF.

If entered into the IVF program, one is under no obligation to complete it. An individual may decide not to complete the program at any time. If this should occur, it would not prevent one from receiving medical care at the Johns Hopkins Medical Institutions.

If you agree to join this study, please signify consent by signing below:

Patient's Signature ⎯⎯⎯⎯⎯⎯⎯⎯⎯ Date ⎯⎯⎯⎯⎯⎯⎯⎯⎯

Witness' Signature ⎯⎯⎯⎯⎯⎯⎯⎯⎯ Date ⎯⎯⎯⎯⎯⎯⎯⎯⎯

I have explained the above to the patient on the date stated on this consent form.

Physician's Signature ⎯⎯⎯⎯⎯⎯⎯⎯⎯ Date ⎯⎯⎯⎯⎯⎯⎯⎯⎯

## INFORMED CONSENT—THE JOHNS HOPKINS HOSPITAL PROGESTERONE INJECTIONS

I understand that my doctors believe my inability to become pregnant or carry a pregnancy may be due to inadequate preparation of the lining of the womb (endometrium) so that the fertilized egg cannot successfully become implanted. Because of this problem I understand that my doctors recommend I receive the medication progesterone in daily injections after ovulation occurs as directed by my doctor. I understand that this medication is to be continued until the menstrual period begins or, if I should become pregnant, it will be continued once pregnancy is confirmed. I understand that the progesterone I will receive is a natural hormone identical to that made by my own body and therefore is unlikely to cause any bad effects to myself or to my baby if I should become pregnant while using this medication.

I further understand that the Food and Drug Administration has advised that medications of this type should not be given to women who may be pregnant since there is evidence that they may cause abnormalities in the baby. The types of abnormalities that have been reported when the mother takes progesterone-like drugs during pregnancy are listed below:

1. Heart defects
2. Anal blockage
3. Abnormalities of bones
4. Abnormal development of brain or spinal cord
5. Vertebral
6. Inguinal hernia
7. Kidney defects
8. Cleft lip or cleft palate
9. Blockage of the swallowing tube
10. Abnormal sex organs
11. Other congenital anomalies not described above

My doctors explained to me that the drugs that caused these abnormalities are synthetic (man-made) drugs whereas the progesterone injections are made from natural progesterone and therefore are no different from the hormones produced by my body and unlikely to cause an increased chance of birth defects in the baby if I get pregnant during its use. I understand that it has not been proven that progesterone is safe and birth defects may occur if I become pregnant while using this medication.

## THE JOHNS HOPKINS IN VITRO FERTILIZATION PROGRAM
### *INFORMED CONSENT: HUMAN EMBRYO CRYOPRESERVATION*

We have been selected as possible participants because we are presently in vitro fertilization (IVF) patients at the Johns Hopkins Institutions. Pre-embryo cryopreservation is available when more than *five* (5) pre-embryos are produced during our IVF treatment cycle. Any pre-embryos developing in excess of five may be cryopreserved as an alternative to transfer. This procedure may benefit us by reducing the probability of multiple births and potential obstetric complications, while also resulting in more opportunities for the initiation of pregnancy with the transfer of pre-embryos developed from frozen-thawed pre-embryos.

Many in vitro laboratories worldwide have demonstrated the ability to cryopreserve human pre-embryos and to establish pregnancy after transfer. Several normal babies have been born subsequent to the transfer of such frozen-thawed pre-embryos. Extensive studies of these human pre-embryos have not demonstrated a significant increase in risk of abnormalities associated with cryopreservation in offspring that had been cryopreserved. We understand that cryopreservation will not eliminate the normal risk of obstetric complications or fetal abnormalities. We understand that cryopreservation does not appear to create an increased risk.

We understand that frozen pre-embryos will not be released from storage for the purpose of intrauterine transfer without the written consents of us both.

We may withdraw our consent and discontinue participation in cryopreservation at any time without prejudice and we understand our pre-embryos will be stored only as long as we are active IVF patients at The Johns Hopkins Hospital Division of Reproductive Endocrinology or until the end of "our normal reproductive years." We have the principal responsibility to decide the disposition of our pre-embryos. We understand that frozen pre-embryos will not be released from storage for the purpose of intrauterine transfer to us without the written consents of us both. In the event of separation or divorce, we understand legal ownership of any stored pre-embryos must be determined in a property settlement and will be released as directed by order of a court of competent jurisdiction. For any reason should we no longer wish to attempt to initiate a pregnancy, we understand we may choose one of three options for our pre-embryos that remain in frozen storage. Our pre-embryos may be:

1. Donated to another willing infertile couple (who will remain unknown to us)
2. Donated for approved research investigation
3. Thawed but not allowed to undergo further development

The possibility of death of one or both prospective parents, or any other unforseen circumstances (such as one prospective parent wishes to remove cryopreserved pre-embryos) that may result in one or neither of us being able to determine the fate of any stored pre-embryos requires that we *indicate our wishes now*. We understand that one of the three decisions listed above must be made, encircled, and initialed by both husband and wife on this form today and written out on the following page.

Storage fees for pre-embryos will be $_____ per month with the first one (1) year fee payable at the time of cryopreservation. Should the transfer of pre-embryos occur prior to the one (1) year period, a refund of the balance will be given. At the end of one (1) year's time, if the pre-embryos have not been transferred, another 1 year fee must be paid. Failure to meet storage fees, or loss of contact with prospective parents for more than two (2) months will result in option three (3) above being carried out.

If the operation of the Johns Hopkins In Vitro Fertilization laboratory discontinues, the couple may have the pre-embryos transferred to another recognized laboratory. However, option three (3) above will be carried out if the couple does not desire the pre-embryos to be transferred at that time, or the couple is not able to be reached within one (1) month's time. No shipping, mailing, or transport of cryopreserved pre-embryos by courier or any means of transportation will be carried out between the Johns Hopkins In Vitro Fertilization laboratory and any other institution, laboratory, or facility.

## Statement

In the event that we are unable to make a decision, we now indicate our desire to have any or all of our pre-embryos in storage:

_____

_____

_____

_____

Husband's Signature _____ Date _____

Wife's Signature _____ Date _____

Any information obtained during these procedures that can be identified with us will remain confidential and will be described to individuals not connected with this project with our written permission only. We understand that photographs or video tapes may be taken of the pre-embryos during the cryopreservation procedures as a permanent record and for possible use at medical meetings or with the lay public for educational purpose. We understand that confidentiality will be maintained. Any new information developed during the course of this investigation that may effect our willingness to continue participation will be provided to us.

We understand that with any technique necessitating mechanical support systems, equipment failure can occur. Neither the Johns Hopkins Institutions nor the Division of Reproductive Endocrinology, its directors, employees, or consultants are to be held liable for any destruction, damage, misuse or improper testing, freezing, maintenance storage, withdrawal, thawing, and/or delivery caused by or resulting from any gross negligence, malfunction of the storage tank, any failure of utilities, any strike, cessation of services, or other labor disturbance, any war, acts of a public enemy, or other disturbance, any fire, wind, earthquake, water, or other acts of God, or the failure of any other laboratory.

We are advised that Johns Hopkins Institutions provide no insurance coverage, compensation plan or free medical care plan to compensate us if we or our pre-embryos are harmed in any way by this cryopreservation procedure.

We understand it is our responsibility to notify the Johns Hopkins In Vitro Fertilization Program Nurse Coordinator of any change in our address and phone number (listed below).

Wife's Signature _____ Date _____

Husband's Signature _____ Date _____

I have explained the above to the subjects on the date stated on this consent form.

Physician's Signature _____ Date _____

# The IVF-ET Procedure

# Physiologic Principles of Induction of Ovulation

Howard A. Zacur and Arnold Goodman

Normal human ovarian follicular development requires an integrated sequence of events involving the coordinated participation of the hypothalamus, pituitary, and ovaries. These events ultimately lead to the release of mature, fertilizable ova from ovarian follicles. In principle, mimicking these events should allow the clinician to induce ovulation resulting in fertilization of a single oocyte without causing ovarian hyperstimulation. An appreciation of the physiologic processes involved in normal ovarian follicular growth and development is essential for the physician using protein and steroid hormones to induce ovulation. A review of the normal physiology of follicular growth and development will therefore be provided prior to discussing various protocols used in ovulation induction.

## HYPOTHALAMIC-PITUITARY INFLUENCE

A relationship between central nervous system activity and pituitary secretion of luteinizing hormone (LH) and follicle stimulating hormone (FSH) was inferred from the classic studies of Smith and Greep (6, 20) who demonstrated that gonadotropin concentrations fell when the pituitary gland was removed and transplanted elsewhere in the body, but rose again when the pituitary was retransplanted beneath the median eminence of the brain. Harris proposed the neurovascular hypothesis that the pituitary is regulated by hypothalamic factors secreted into the hypophysial portal vessels (8). This neurovascular relationship between the hypothalamus and the pituitary was further defined in 1971 by researchers in the laboratories of Schally and Guillemin who isolated and characterized first thyrotropin releasing hormone (TRH) then gonadotropin releasing hormone (GnRH), also known as LH releasing hormone (3, 15). GnRH is a decapeptide found in high concentration in the median eminence of the brain that stimulates the release of LH and FSH from the pituitary gland. A cloned complementary DNA sequence encoding human GnRH has now been utilized by Nikolics and colleagues to detect a GnRH precursor protein (17). In mice a deletion in the GnRH gene has been identified and believed to be responsible for the hypogonadal condition found in the hereditary hypogonadal mouse (14). This condition mimics the human hypogonadal state known as Kallmann's syndrome (11) characterized by olfactory bulb agenesis, anosmia, and hypogonadism. This clinical disorder is more frequently seen in men than women. Gonadal stimulation using exogenously administered GnRH in these patients has resulted in spermatogenesis or ovulation.

Following its discovery, initial attempts to induce ovulation with GnRH succeeded only when GnRH was given as a bolus after follicular development had been maximally stimulated with gonadotropins (12). Administration of GnRH as a daily injection failed to induce ovulation if prior gonadotropin stimulation of the ovary had not occurred. These initial attempts to induce ovulation with GnRH did not represent a failure to have identified the appropriate hormone responsible for pituitary LH and FSH secretion, but rather a failure in how to administer GnRH appropriately. Knobil and colleagues studied the regulation of gonadotropin secretion in adult female rhesus monkeys that had undergone bilateral radiofrequency lesions of the arcuate region of the medial basal hypothalamus. This procedure abolished secretion of endogenous GnRH and re-

The authors wish to acknowledge Dr. Arlene Morales and Dr. Sue Ellen Carpenter, Department of Gynecology and Obstetrics, for their assistance in the preparation of this manuscript.

sulted in lowered LH and FSH levels and loss of menstrual cycles in the monkeys (13, 18). On receiving unvarying, intravenous pulses of synthetic GnRH at hourly intervals, normal gonadotropin levels and menstrual cycles were reestablished (16). This information from non-human primate studies provided the rationale for administering GnRH in pulsatile form to anovulatory human patients. When given in this manner, ovulation induction with GnRH has been quite successful (23).

Knobil and colleagues initially argued that the release of pituitary LH resulted from an unvarying frequency and constant amplitude of release of hypothalamic GnRH and that GnRH was therefore permissive to pituitary LH secretion (13). That LH pulses during the human luteal phase exhibit greater amplitude and reduced frequency when compared with LH pulses during the follicular phase challenges this action (22). This change in pulsatility may reflect progesterone modulation of hypothalamic GnRH release. As a consequence of these experimental findings, use of GnRH to induce ovulation and restore fertility may require modification during the luteal phase of the induced cycle, or supplementation with either human chorionic gonadotropin (hCG) or progesterone to maintain an adequate luteal phase (2).

## INTRAOVARIAN FOLLICULAR REGULATION

Follicular growth and development within the human ovary may be defined in terms of recruitment, selection, and dominance as described by Goodman and Hodgen (5). The number of human oocytes present in the ovaries is fixed at birth, and ovarian function remains largely quiescent until puberty. An explanation for the restrained ovarian activity prior to puberty remains elusive but is felt to be due to diminished pituitary secretion of gonadotropins, which in turn reflects diminished hypothalamic release of GnRH.

At menarche the human ovary contains hundreds of thousands of primordial follicles, which are azonal oocytes, each surrounded by a single layer of flattened granulosa cells (Fig. 7-1). During each menstrual cycle, groups of primordial follicles leave the resting state and become growing primary follicles; this process appears to be gonadotropin independent but may be enhanced by FSH. Follicular development past preantral stages requires gonadotropins. In brief, from data obtained from experiments performed in rats, granulosa cells in primary follicles possess FSH but not LH receptors. In response to FSH stimulation, more FSH receptors appear on the granulosa cells. In addition in response to FSH stimulation, the granulosa cells produce an enzyme that can convert the androgens androstenedione and testosterone to estrone and estradiol, respectively. LH receptors are not found in granulosa cells taken from preantral follicles but are found on theca cells, which interestingly lack FSH receptors. Stimulation of the theca cells by LH results in the secretion by these cells of androstenedione and testosterone, which diffuses across the basement membrane and into the avascular follicle as depicted in Fig. 7-2. This hormonal process has been described as the "two-cell theory."

In response to both LH and FSH stimulation, primary follicles enlarge by increasing the numbers of granulosa cells. Increasing amounts of estradiol are then secreted by the enlarging follicle into the peripheral circulation as the increased numbers of granulosa cells provide more aromatase converting androgens to estrogens. Eventually a very large 2-cm diameter follicle with a fluid-filled antrum is formed, which is called a *preovulatory* or *graafian follicle* containing the oocyte that will be released at ovulation following the midcycle LH surge.

### Recruitment

Presumably the conversion of primordial to primary follicles is a continuous process enhanced by FSH but capable of proceeding as a result of local intraovarian control mechanisms that are not well understood. Recruitment begins

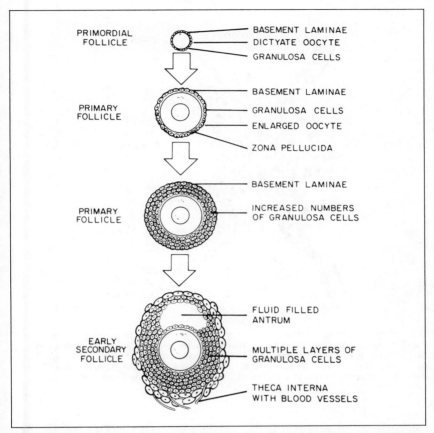

**Fig. 7-1. Follicular development sequence from primordial to early secondary follicle. (Modified from G. F. Erickson. Normal ovarian function. *Clin. Obstet. Gynecol.* 21:31, 1978. With permission.)**

in earnest when this available pool of primary follicles is stimulated by FSH to begin further development. From the elegant studies of Hodgen alone and with Goodman (5, 9) using the subhuman primate, it is now clear that follicular development from primary to preovulatory stage requires at least 14 days. Furthermore, it appears that this process is not significantly influenced by events occurring during the previous menstrual cycle(s). Continuation of the recruitment process requires sufficient exposure by the ovaries and their pool of primary follicles to FSH and LH. Pituitary gonadotropins, although required for follicular growth and development, are not directing these events, which are in fact being controlled by intraovarian factors.

### Selection
*Selection* refers to the limitation, by the ovary early in the follicular phase, to one growing follicle that will be solely responsible for releasing the oocyte. Surprisingly, selection occurs quite early, before the sixth day of the follicular phase. Identification of a dominant follicle in the nonhuman primate at this early date was confirmed indirectly by Hodgen and Goodman (5, 9) who detected

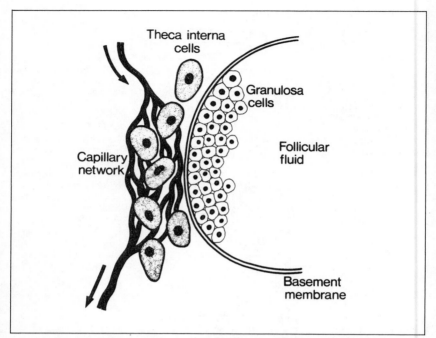

Fig. 7-2. Theca cells stimulated by LH from capillary network secreting androgens that serve as precursors in granulosa cell estrogen synthesis. (From D. T. Baird. Reproductive Hormones in Reproduction. In C. R. Austin and R. V. Shorts (eds.), *Reproduction in Mammals* (Vol. 3). New York: Cambridge University Press, 1972. With permission.)

asymmetric ovarian vein estradiol concentrations. This indirect evidence was most important since, histologically, the dominant follicle could not be detected in the group of primary follicles in either ovary at this time. It remains unclear as to the precise criteria used by the ovary to "select" its dominant follicle. Of course this selection process may be overridden by administration of exogenous human menopausal gonadotropins, but to be maximally effective these gonadotropins should be given prior to the time that dominance is normally attained.

## Dominance

*Dominance* is the term used to describe the influence exerted by the selected graafian follicle to ensure its exclusive continued development to the detriment of other growing follicles in the ipsilateral and contralateral ovary. An accurate explanation for this mechanism does not currently exist. Current theories rely on suggesting an alteration in FSH receptors induced by local paracrine or autocrine factors in the ovary. This might include some of the recently described ovarian growth factors, such as activin or transforming growth factor, which could modulate the end-organ response of FSH (21). As previously mentioned the selection of the dominant follicle occurs in the subhuman primate between days 5–7 of the follicular phase. After that time the dominant follicle so selected exerts a negative influence on further development of other follicles. Interestingly although the ovarian selection process may be overridden by the use of exogenous gonadotropins, reversal or override of the "dominance" phase is not easily attained. This was reported by DiZerega and Hodgen using nonhuman primates (4). In their study, human menopausal gonadotropin (hMG) administration did not stimulate further follicle development after the dominant follicle had been selected.

## OVULATION

Following the selection of the dominant follicle, its continued growth to the exclusion of other follicles results in the formation of a large preovulatory or graafian follicle existing usually around the fourteenth day of the menstrual cycle. At this point, in response to a large midcycle surge in estradiol coming from the dominant preovulatory follicle, a large release of pituitary LH takes place, resulting in oocyte release 24–36 hours later. The midcycle LH surge is extremely important not only in triggering the process of ovulation but in causing maturation of the oocyte. Throughout follicular growth, the oocyte has remained arrested in the diplotene stage of the first meiotic prophase. It is surrounded by tightly adhering granulosa cells called *cumulus cells*. If aspirated from the follicle, the oocyte at this stage is incapable of undergoing fertilization. Following the LH surge, the oocyte completes its first meiotic division, extrudes the first polar body, and becomes capable of being fertilized. Resumption of meiosis is characterized by breakdown of the oocyte nucleus (germinal vesicle breakdown). This process may occur in vitro spontaneously when oocytes are removed from the follicle or may occur in vivo following a gonadotropin surge. Cumulus cells surrounding the immature oocyte form tight layers. These layers expand as the oocyte matures and finally disperse into loosely adherent cells.

Biochemical processes involved in ovulation itself are under active investigation by several research laboratories. In brief, the LH surge is followed by changes in blood flow in vessels surrounding the preovulatory follicle, within which the follicle secretion of proteins, steroids, enzymes, and prostaglandins occurs. Eventually plasminogen becomes activated to form plasmin, which initiates a cascade of enzymatic digestion of follicle wall collagen, by activating collagenolytic enzymes eventually resulting in oocyte release.

## CORPUS LUTEUM FORMATION

After ovulation, granulosa and theca cells within the follicle become luteinized. These cells secrete the steroid progesterone, and increased progesterone concentrations can be detected during the periovulatory interval. Peripheral progesterone concentrations are normally lower than 3 ng/ml during the follicle phase of the cycle. The ability of granulosa cells to luteinize is acquired after LH receptors appear, allowing these cells to respond to the midcycle LH surge. Following oocyte release the basement membrane of the follicle dissolves, and, in response to a presumed angiogenic signal, vessels invade the reorganizing follicle. Cells of the newly forming corpus luteum are derived from both the granulosa and theca. In the formed corpus luteum, large luteal cells are derived from the *granulosa* and small luteal cells are derived from the *theca*. Continued secretion of progesterone from luteal cells requires LH.

Secretion of progesterone is important in order to effect changes in the endometrium required for implantation. Corpus luteum progesterone production has also been suggested as an important factor in inhibiting follicular growth and development during the luteal phase. Progesterone may do this by suppressing follicular growth within the same and opposite ovaries. Alternatively, other as yet undiscovered substances may be responsible for this. Increased release of inhibin to lower FSH levels or release by the dominant follicle of a follicle regulatory protein to depress estrogen production by other follicles is another alternative explanation.

The principles of ovulation induction are a direct result of understanding the normal processes of follicular development and ovulation. These include follicular selection, recruitment, and dominance as well as ovulation and corpus luteum formation. Under normal conditions these events occur smoothly as a result of the coordinated interplay among hypothalamus, pituitary, and ovary. Ovulation induction implies that normal extra- and intraovarian regulatory mechanisms will be superceded by exogenously administered substances. These might include steroid hormone receptor antagonists, e.g., clomiphene citrate, hypothalamic peptides, e.g., GnRH and analogs, as well as pituitary glycoproteins, e.g., LH and FSH. Efficacious use of these agents should be maximized by adhering to the principles of follicular maturation previously discussed.

## Clomiphene Citrate

This is a triphenylethylene derivative containing a chloride anion and an aminoalkoxyl group. Despite the synthesis and use of the drug since the 1950s, its precise mode of action remains unclear. Clomiphene citrate exists in either a cis or trans form with the cis form being biologically more active as an estrogen agonist. Commercially available clomiphene citrate contains both the cis and trans forms in equal amounts. Use of this drug is believed to prevent estrogen receptor replenishment in cells of the hypothalamic pituitary axis. As a consequence, increased pituitary secretion of gonadotropins occurs, stimulating follicular growth.

Use of clomiphene citrate to induce ovulation will be of benefit to anovulatory patients with heightened endogenous estrogenic activity, e.g., "polycystic ovarian disease (PCO) patients," ovulatory patients requiring improved timing of ovulation or ovulatory patients undergoing ovulation induction with hMG during in vitro fertilization (IVF) cycles (1).

Use of clomiphene citrate will therefore result in increased gonadotropin secretion that will override the ovarian regulatory mechanisms responsible for follicle recruitment, selection, and dominance. As a result, more than one preovulatory follicle may be stimulated, thereby increasing the chances of multiple pregnancy. Use of clomiphene citrate may also result in estrogen antagonism at the ovary, uterus, and cervix, in addition to the hypothalamus. Consequently, poor follicular and oocyte development with diminished endometrial progesterone receptors and decreased cervical mucus secretion may result. Ovulation induction protocols for IVF using clomiphene citrate usually do so in conjunction with hMGs, and these protocols will be discussed at the conclusion of the section on hMG ovulation induction.

## Human Gonadotropin Therapy

Gonadotropins extracted from the urine of menopausal women may be administered to induce ovulation. hMG preparations contain both LH and FSH biologic activities in equal amounts. Usually both FSH and LH are required to induce ovulation since LH will stimulate androgen production from theca cells and FSH will stimulate aromatase production from granulosa cells. Aromatase will convert androgens to estrogen. Success in using hMG requires that it be given at the appropriate time and dose. hMG is less effective in causing follicular recruitment and growth if given after selection of the dominant follicle (day 5–7) (4). Therefore in ovulatory women given hMG as part of an IVF protocol, early onset of hMG use is important. Dosage of hMG is by necessity individualized depending on the patient's responses. Dosage schedules may be fixed, e.g., two ampules per day, or variable. In variable schedules, higher to lower (e.g., four then three then two ampules per day) or lower to higher regimens (e.g., two then three then four ampules per day) may be used. Monitored parameters include daily plasma estradiol concentrations, changes in vaginal epithelium and cervical mucus, and ultrasonographic changes in numbers and sizes of developing follicles. In general hMG will be stopped when estradiol concentrations are around or above 600 pg/ml, following a shift of biologic parameters, i.e., increased numbers of pyknotic cells in vaginal smears and increased cervical mucus production and a follicle at least 18 mm in diameter (10). Completion of the ovulation induction protocol requires administration of 10,000 units of hCG.

Empiric use of hCG is required as an LH surge substitute to complete oocyte maturation and initiate luteinization and ovulation. Patient responses to this ovulation induction scheme may vary significantly, but once an individual response pattern is established, it will be repeated if the ovulation induction protocol remains unchanged. In anovulatory individuals sufficient doses of hMG to raise the plasma estradiol concentration to 1000 pg/ml may be required (19). Risk of ovarian hyperstimulation is reduced if estradiol concentrations are kept lower than 1500 pg/ml (7).

### hMG in Combination with Pure FSH, GnRH Analog, or Clomiphene

Centers utilizing hMG in IVF ovulation induction protocols have combined administration of hMG with other agents in efforts to improve response. Use of pure FSH coupled with hMG early in the induction protocol has been helpful in increasing the estradiol concentration in poor responders. Usually two ampules of pure FSH are given with two ampules of hMG as divided doses for the initial 2 days of the ovulation induction. In some programs clomiphene citrate (100 mg) is given from days 5–9 and hMG begun on day 8 onward. This protocol may improve the response to clomiphene only or may reduce the total number of hMG ampules needed if only hMG were to be given.

A most recent change in ovulation induction protocols has included the use of GnRH analogs. These have been given either to improve patient response to hMG or the timing of ovulation induction for later oocyte retrieval. Various combinational protocols have been employed using long-term use, short-term use, initiation at onset of menses, or in midluteal phase, as discussed in detail in Chapter 8.

### Complications

Primary complications from the ovulation induction protocols described include ovarian hyperstimulation, multiple gestation, and increased spontaneous abortion rates. Risk of ovarian hyperstimulation is minimized by carefully monitoring the plasma estradiol concentration and the ovaries by ultrasound. Keeping the estradiol concentration lower than 1500 pg/ml will greatly limit the risk of hyperstimulation. If doubt exists as to whether hyperstimulation will occur, the dose of hCG is withheld. Hyperstimulation is extremely unlikely in the absence of hCG. Risk of multiple gestation has been quoted as 5% for clomiphene citrate and 20% for hMG when these drugs are used solely for ovulation induction and not as part of an IVF protocol. In non-IVF cycles, risk of multiple pregnancy may be reduced somewhat by carefully monitoring the ovaries by ultrasound and withholding hCG if too many follicles are seen. In IVF protocols maximum-oocyte retrieval is desirable, and multiple pregnancy rates will be determined to a degree by the number of embryos transferred.

Increased rates of spontaneous abortion following conceptions induced by clomiphene citrate or hMG have been previously reported. Explanations for this have included estrogenic deprivation of the oocyte following clomiphene induction of ovulation or luteal phase deficiency following either clomiphene or hMG ovulation induction. Diagnosis of luteal phase deficiency is facilitated by use of the timed endometrial biopsy, and treatment has consisted of exogenous progesterone administration. During IVF cycles, concerns for luteal phase deficiency have been raised not only because of the use of hMG itself but because follicle aspiration may remove significant numbers of granulosa cells, resulting in diminished numbers of luteinized granulosa cells or "large" corpora luteal cells with a corresponding decline in progesterone secretion. Counter arguments have included the fact that hMG-stimulated ovaries provide more than one corpus luteum, which should provide sufficient progesterone concentrations.

The normal changes in follicular growth and development have been reviewed and the interaction of the hypothalamus, pituitary, and ovary in this process described. With this knowledge a better understanding should exist as to how ovulation-inducing drugs such as clomiphene citrate and hMG may be used to maximum effect with minimal risk.

## REFERENCES

1. Adashi, E. Y. Clomiphene citrate initiated ovulated: A clinical update. *Semin. Reprod. Endocrinol.* (4)3:255, 1986.
2. Berger, N. G., and Zacur, H. A. Exogenous progesterone for luteal support following gonadotropin-releasing hormone ovulation induction: Case report. *Fertil. Steril.* 44:133, 1985.
3. Burgus, R., et al. Primary structure of the hypothalamic luteinizing hormone releasing factor (LRF) of ovine origin. *Proc. Natl. Acad. Sci. U.S.A.* 69:278, 1972.
4. DiZerega, G. S., and Hodgen, G. D. The primate ovarian cycle: Suppression of human menopausal gonadotropin-induced follicular growth in the presence of the dominant follicle. *J. Clin. Endocrinol. Metab.* 50:819, 1980.
5. Goodman, A. L., and Hodgen, G. D. The ovarian triad of the primate menstrual cycle. *Recent Prog. Horm. Res.* 39:1, 1983.
6. Greep, R. O. Functional pituitary grafts in rats. *Proc. Soc. Exp. Biol. Med.* 34:754, 1936.
7. Hanning, R. V., et al. Plasma estradiol is superior to ultrasound and urinary estradiol glucuronide as a predictor of ovarian hyperstimulation during induction of ovulation with menotropins. *Fertil. Steril.* 40:31, 1983.
8. Harris, G. W. *Neural Control of the Pituitary Gland.* Baltimore: Williams & Wilkins, 1955.
9. Hodgen, G. D. The dominant ovarian follicle. *Fertil. Steril.* 38:281, 1982.
10. Jones, G. E. S. Update in in vitro fertilization. *Endocrin. Rev.* (5)1:62, 1984.
11. Kallmann, F. J., Schoenfeld, W. A., and Barrera, S. E. The genetic aspects of primary eunuchoidism. *Am. J. Ment. Defic.* 48:203, 1948.
12. Kastin, A. J. et al. Ovulation confirmed by pregnancy after infusion of porcine LH-RH. *J. Clin. Endocrinol. Metab.* 33:980, 1971.
13. Knobil, E., et al. Control of the Rhesus monkey menstrual cycle: Permissive role of hypothalamic gonadotropin releasing hormone. *Science* 207:1371, 1980.
14. Mason, A. J., et al. A deletion truncating the gonadotropin releasing hormone gene is responsible for hypogonadism in the hpg mouse. *Science* 234:1366, 1986.
15. Matsuo, H., et al. Structure of the porcine LH and FSH releasing hormone: I. The proposed amino acid sequence. *Biochem. Biophys. Res. Commun.* 43:1334, 1971.
16. Nakai, Y., et al. On the sites of negative and positive feedback actions of estradiol in the control of gonadotropin secretion in the Rhesus monkey. *Endocrinology* 102:1008, 1978.
17. Nikolics, K., et al. A prolactin-inhibiting factor within the precursor for human gonadotropin-releasing hormone. *Nature* 316:511, 1985.
18. Plant, T. M., et al. The arcuate nucleus and the control of gonadotropin and prolactin secretion in the female Rhesus monkey (Macaca mulatta) *Endocrinology* 102:52, 1978.
19. Schwartz, M., and Jewelewicz, K. The use of gonadotropins for induction of ovulation. *Fertil. Steril.* 35:3, 1981.
20. Smith, P. E. Postponed pituitary homotransplants into the region of the hypophysial portal circulation of hypophysectomized female rats. *Endocrinology* 73:793, 1963.
21. Tonetta, S. A., and DiZerega, G. S. Intragonadal regulation of follicular maturation. *Endocr. Rev.* 10:205, 1989.
22. Yen, S. S. C., et al. Ultradian fluctuations of gonadotropins. In M. Ferin et al. (eds.), *Biorhythms and Human Reproduction.* New York: Wiley, 1974. P. 203.
23. Zacur, H. A. Ovulation induction with gonadotropin releasing hormone. *Fertil. Steril.* 44:435, 1985.

# Follicular Maturation and Monitoring for IVF-ET

John S. Hesla

The first successful in vitro fertilization (IVF) pregnancy arose from the fertilization of a single oocyte recovered from a dominant follicle in a natural menstrual cycle (85). Further experience with this new technology revealed that pregnancy rates were improved by increasing the number of embryos available for transfer through controlled ovarian hyperstimulation (94). Disadvantages associated with the use of the spontaneous menstrual cycle included the need for frequent testing for the luteinizing hormone (LH) surge as well as a lack of flexibility in scheduling the oocyte retrieval for the patient, surgeon, and laboratory personnel. As a result, the vast majority of IVF programs have abandoned follicular aspiration in an unstimulated cycle for protocols utilizing ovulation induction.

*The aims of ovarian hyperstimulation in IVF are to*

1. Promote the development of a relatively synchronous cohort of follicles. Sonographic evidence of a close approximation of follicular size facilitates the appropriate timing of human chorionic gonadotropin (hCG) administration and oocyte retrieval.
2. Collect multiple, mature oocytes that have the capacity to fertilize, cleave, and initiate a viable pregnancy.
3. Achieve endometrial development that will support embryonic implantation and growth.
4. Minimize the cycle cancellation rate due to poor parameters of follicular response.
5. Maximize cost efficiency of medications and monitoring.

Studies in primates clearly indicate that an injection of hCG given at an inappropriate time during ovarian stimulation will result in an abnormally matured oocyte that does not have the potential for normal embryonic development (94). Although immature oocytes can be matured in vitro, these eggs rarely lead to pregnancy. Hence, accurate clinical assessment of oocyte maturity is critical to the success of an IVF program.

Follicular development up to the small antral stage in women occurs over a period of approximately 85 days and is unaffected by fluctuations in levels of pituitary gonadotropins (30). The growing follicles are likely recruited in a random manner from a pool of primordial oocytes, and, as a result, some asynchrony of development exists among the cohort of follicles. Current theories propose that the selection of follicles destined for more advanced maturation occurs during and shortly after the end of the luteal phase of the antecedent menstrual cycle (33) (Fig. 8-1). Corpus luteum regression is associated with a fall in estradiol and progesterone levels and a decline in the negative feedback of these hormones on gonadotropin secretion. As the FSH concentration rises above that threshold necessary to stimulate the aromatase enzyme system of the granulosa cell, development proceeds beyond the 4-mm stage in select follicles (3) (Fig. 8-2). Asymmetry in estradiol production by the two ovaries can be measured by day 5 of the spontaneous cycle due to the recruitment of a single dominant follicle destined for ovulation (13). Increased secretion of estradiol, inhibin, and other factors by the developing follicle suppresses pituitary gonadotropin release, which in turn inhibits maturation of the secondary follicles. The granulosa cells in these smaller follicles become atretic due to the lack of follicle stimulating hormone (FSH) stimulation. In contrast, the high estradiol concen-

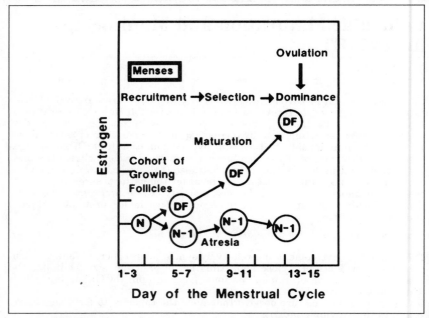

Fig. 8-1. Time course for recruitment, selection, and ovulation of the dominant ovarian follicle in the spontaneous menstrual cycle. (From G. D. Hodgen. The dominant ovarian follicle. *Fertil. Steril.* 38:281, 1982. With permission.)

tration within the dominant follicle markedly enhances local FSH and LH action, thereby allowing this follicle to continue to develop in an FSH-deficient milieu (74).

With ovulation induction via administration of clomiphene citrate (CC, Clomid, Serophene) or human menopausal gonadotropins (hMG, Pergonal), the threshold gonadotropin requirements of several follicles in the early stages of development are exceeded, allowing the recruitment of codominant follicles (Fig. 8-3). This stimulation may rescue large follicles in the early stages of atresia through a recovered growth ability of the granulosa cells (70). When ovarian stimulation is initiated on cycle day 3, the recruited follicles are already at different developmental stages and continue to lack total synchrony as they mature. The majority of patients undergoing ovulation induction with hMG fail to experience an endogenous midcycle surge of FSH and LH despite supraphysiologic concentrations of estradiol (45). This alteration in normal feedback mechanisms usually permits a cohort of follicles to develop to maturity and avert premature luteinization by rising LH levels.

The magnitude of follicular response to hMG or CC administration can be assessed by different means. Sonography is commonly used to determine the follicular number, dimensions, and position on the ovary. Blood estradiol and urinary estrogen concentrations are a systemic reflection of the endocrine microenvironment of the selected cohort. Monitoring of changes in vaginal cytology, cervical mucus, plasma progesterone, and LH levels may be advantageous in estimating the normalcy of follicular response.

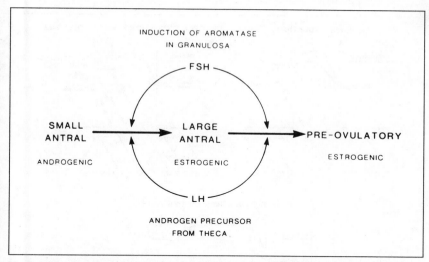

INDUCTION OF AROMATASE
IN GRANULOSA

FSH

SMALL
ANTRAL

LARGE
ANTRAL

PRE-OVULATORY

ANDROGENIC

ESTROGENIC

ESTROGENIC

LH

ANDROGEN PRECURSOR
FROM THECA

**Fig. 8-2. Development of follicles. Both FSH and LH play a role in increasing the capacity of the developing follicle to produce estradiol. (From D. T. Baird. A model for follicular selection and ovulation: lessons from superovulation.** *J. Steroid Biochem.* **27:15, 1987. With permission.)**

## SONOGRAPHY

Sonographic scanning is begun in the early follicular phase on the day of initiation of ovarian stimulation in order to assess the structural state of the ovary. Follicular development suggestive of early selection of a dominant follicle precludes hMG or CC administration, particularly if confirmed by an elevated baseline estradiol level. In addition, a large ovarian cyst may be considered a contraindication to ovulation induction because of its potential responsiveness to gonadotropin therapy. An alternative to cycle cancellation in such instances is a transvaginal aspiration of the cyst via sonographic guidance prior to proceeding with ovulation induction. Pelvic sonography with a vaginal transducer has replaced the transvesical-transabdominal approach in our institution due to its superior imaging and improved patient comfort. Repeat sonographic scanning after the initial study is unnecessary until the patient manifests a biologic response to the stimulation therapy based on physical examination findings or estrogen assay. The scans are repeated daily thereafter up to the day of oocyte retrieval.

With accumulation of secretory products of the growing follicle in the intracellular spaces of the granulosa layer, the follicle enters the antral stage of development and becomes sonographically visible as an echolucent cyst within the ovary (41) (Fig. 8-4). Because of the potential errors in imaging technique and interpretation of results, an average follicle diameter should be calculated from the transverse, longitudinal, and anterior-posterior measurements. Follicles in the hyperstimulated ovary are frequently compressed by adjacent follicles, resulting in an asymmetric shape. Mathematic determination of total follicular volume of each ovary is another useful method of monitoring follicular growth. The range of follicular volume produced by ovarian hyperstimulation is wide, probably owing to the recruitment of follicles into antral growth at variable times during the induction. Most observers have found a linear increase in follicular diameter during the last 5 days of ovulation (41). The growth rate

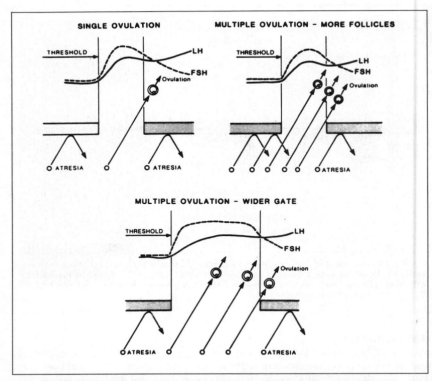

Fig. 8-3. Baird's model for selection of the dominant follicle in the early follicular phase of the menstrual cycle. Multiple ovulation may be stimulated by providing a greater number of synchronous follicles or by lengthening the time during which the level of FSH remains elevated above the threshold necessary for development beyond the small antral stage. (From D. T. Baird. A model for follicular selection and ovulation: lessons from superovulation. *J. Steroid Biochem.* 27:15, 1987. With permission.)

during this period ranges from 1.5–3.1 mm per 24 hours. Vargyas and colleagues reported a mean daily follicular growth rate of 2.4 mm per 24 hours and a preovulatory mean diameter of the lead follicle of 22.1 ± 0.4 mm in CC/hMG-treated cycles (91); these figures approximate those measured in the spontaneous ovulatory cycle. A slower growth rate may reflect inadequate granulosa cell stimulation by the dose of gonadotropin administered. Oocyte maturity is more difficult to predict in stimulated versus unstimulated cycles because the cohort of dominant follicles in the former is asynchronous in size and functional maturation. The relative contribution of an individual follicle to the peripheral pool of estradiol may fluctuate over time (43). In addition, the individual follicle contributes less to peripheral estradiol levels in multifollicular cycles than in monofollicular cycles (19). Studies have reported either a positive correlation or little correlation of the estrogen concentration with mean follicular volume. With multiple follicular development, estradiol levels are more closely associated with the total follicular volume than merely the follicular diameter of the dominant follicle (35, 91). Hence, the number of developing antral follicles must be considered when assessing the patient response to the stimulatory agent. Multiple small follicles may secrete estradiol amounts equivalent to that of a single large

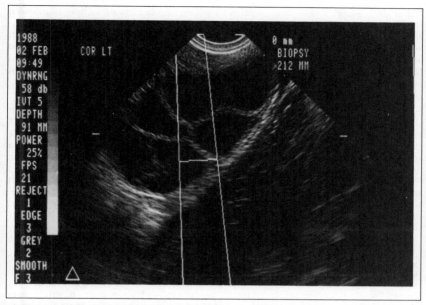

**Fig. 8-4. Vaginal sonographic image of multiple preovulatory follicles. Parallel lines represent pathway boundaries of needle guide for follicular puncture.**

follicle. Sonographic findings are particularly helpful in such instances in determining the appropriate timing of hCG administration.

Nevertheless, the size of the follicle alone does not provide a completely reliable estimate of the oocyte's ability to be fertilized and cleave. Mature oocytes have been retrieved from follicles ranging in size from 1.5–3.0 cm in diameter (35, 42). Most studies have suggested that the majority of normal pregnancies arise from average lead follicular diameters of 1.7–2.3 cm (68, 76). To achieve this size, approximately 6 days of active follicular growth are required as reflected by rising blood estradiol concentrations (50). Some variation in follicular maturity may exist at any given sonographic size, depending on the stimulation regimen used. Gonadotropin-stimulated follicles are smaller at the preovulatory stage than follicles growing under the influence of CC (38); however, pituitary suppression with gonadotropin releasing hormone (GnRH) agonists before and during menotropin ovarian stimulation results in a less mature oocyte at an equivalent follicular size than that obtained via administration of hMG alone (62).

Oocyte distribution based on follicular size has revealed a high percentage of empty follicles and a low percentage of preovulatory and fractured zona oocytes from very small follicles (83). Follicles less than 2.5 cc in volume or approximately 1.5 cm in diameter are more likely to contain immature ova and thus result in a lower possibility that aspiration will yield an embryo for transfer. Even if a cleaving embryo is replaced, the pregnancy outcome in this group remains poor as compared to oocytes originating from larger follicles (67, 83). It may be that the capacity to undergo meiotic maturation in response to hCG is acquired earlier than full cytoplasmic maturity, leading to limitations in developmental capacity of these oocytes.

Other data suggest that those cycles in which the dominant follicle is allowed to grow beyond 2.3 cm are associated with a higher rate of polyspermic fertilization (6). The spontaneous abortion rate is the highest in the patient population with the greatest mean volume of follicles prior to aspiration. Although the oocytes that give rise to successful pregnancies are obtained from follicles containing a high concentration of estradiol, the most estrogenic follicle among a cohort may not be the largest in size (95).

Sonographic imaging may provide additional information of diagnostic significance if performed the day after hCG administration. Structural changes within the follicle during the periovulatory time period may be apparent. A cumulus echo has been observed in over 23% of normal cycles and may reflect oocyte maturity (41). These echoes are presumably due to clumps or sheets of granulosa cells that have detached from the follicular wall. A decrease in mean follicular diameter by 2 mm or more on the day after hCG administration is associated with a low oocyte recovery and fertilization rate, lower cleavage rate, and a high incidence of polyspermic fertilization (6). Premature ovulation prior to the scheduled time of follicular puncture may be diagnosed by disappearance of the follicle, increased echogenicity of the luteinizing cyst, and the presence of free fluid near the ovary and in the cul de sac (31).

## ESTROGEN MEASUREMENT

Rapid follicular development up to the graafian follicle stage has been reported to occur over a 4–5 day period in natural cycles as well as during ovarian stimulation cycles (36). The corresponding changes in steroidogenesis are reflected by an exponential increase in peripheral estrogen from basal to preovulatory peak levels. Hence, daily monitoring of plasma estradiol or total urinary estrogen is of particular merit in assessing the hormonal responsiveness of a developing cohort of follicles. A baseline estradiol level of greater than 100 pg/ml is suggestive of follicular activity by endogenous gonadotropin stimulation. Introduction of hMG or CC in such instances would likely lead to a marked asynchronism in development with rapid enlargement of a single dominant follicle. Ovarian stimulation should be postponed in these patients. Estrogen assays may also provide important information regarding the appropriate dose of hMG for patients undergoing induction. Low estradiol values on 2 or more consecutive days should signal the clinician to increase the amount of gonadotropin administered in order to achieve optimal folliculogenesis; however, a plateau in estradiol concentration during the preovulatory stage of stimulation may precede an impending LH surge (6).

Healthy, normally cycling women of similar weights may have highly variable ovarian responses to a uniform regimen of hMG; however, the response of the individual is typically repetitive when equivalent doses of menotropins are given in subsequent cycles (40). Very low or high estradiol growth rates are associated with a significantly greater likelihood of missed oocyte recovery or fertilization failure, or both. Altering the dose of hMG administered in subsequent stimulation cycles in these patients usually fails to change the number of large preovulatory follicles that develop (8). Nevertheless, the magnitude of the ovarian response may be significantly modified by varying the dose of hMG in high-responder patients. This dose-response correlation is markedly diminished in poor-responding patients. Increasing the dose of hMG in low responders may merely promote the development of small follicles containing oocytes that are unlikely to lead to conception (46) from day 8 onward. The dominant follicles of the hyporesponding patient may be optimally stimulated by low doses of hMG.

The estradiol response pattern associated with the highest pregnancy rate is that in which a progressive rise in estrogen secretion occurs during the course of hMG stimulation, a continued rise between the last menotropin dose and the receipt of hCG, and a further estrogen elevation on the day following the hCG injection (46). Similar results have been demonstrated in CC/hMG-stimulated

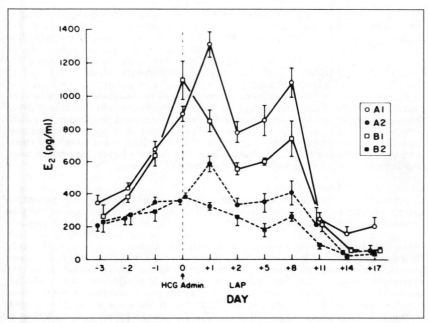

Fig. 8-5. Comparison of four patterns of estradiol response (mean ± SEM) to hMG/hCG stimulation. *Group $A_1$* — estradiol >500 pg/ml on day 0; estradiol levels increase on day +1. *Group $A_2$* — estradiol <500 pg/ml on day 0; estradiol levels increase on day +1. *Group $B_1$* — estradiol >500 pg/ml on day 0; estradiol levels decrease on day +1. *Group $B_2$* — estradiol <500 pg/ml on day 0; estradiol levels decrease on day +1. A significantly higher pregnancy rate was achieved in women with response pattern A. (From N. Laufer et al. The association between preovulatory serum 17 β estradiol pattern and conception in human menopausal gonadotropin-human chorionic gonadotropin stimulation. *Fertil. Steril.* 46:73, 1986. With permission.)

cycles. A drop in serum estradiol prior to hCG administration suggests that luteinization or atresia of the more advanced follicles has spontaneously commenced in response to the development of a threshold level of LH. Polyspermic penetration of the oocyte is more likely when estradiol levels plateau or decline prior to hCG (6). Fewer cleaving oocytes are obtained in stimulation cycles characterized by a fall in estradiol on the day of hCG or the day after hCG. Nevertheless, a plateau in serum estradiol after hCG administration is not associated with a decline in fertilization or cleavage (6). The estradiol response pattern with the poorest prognosis is characterized by a peak estradiol of less than 500 pg/ml and a lack of rise of estrogen after hCG (47) (Fig. 8-5). This perimenopausal, low-response pattern has been associated with an elevated basal serum FSH level as measured on day 3 of the cycle and is positively correlated with advanced patient age (80).

Patients who exhibit a very rapid rise of circulating estradiol in response to ovarian stimulation display the multifollicular response pattern. More than 12 follicles may develop in such patients by the time of oocyte retrieval. These individuals typically have a higher basal LH-FSH ratio than women who manifest moderate- or low-response patterns (64). Estrogen levels must be closely correlated with follicular size to accurately assess oocyte maturity for timing of hCG.

Cancellation of ovulation induction or follicular aspiration should be strongly considered for those patients who fail to demonstrate a significant rise in estradiol concentration after 5 days of hMG therapy or in patients whose estradiol values fall during the final stages of stimulation. Poor estrogen production is generally associated with the development of fewer than two preovulatory follicles of favorable size for IVF. An estradiol value greater than 3000 pg/ml at the time of hCG administration is associated with a significant incidence of ovarian hyperstimulation syndrome, the major serious complication of ovulation induction by gonadotropins (62). This risk is also greater in patients with a fewer number of mature follicles and a relative increased proportion of small follicles on the day of hCG. Follicular aspiration has been postulated to have some protective effect by emptying the large- and medium-sized follicles of their contents of follicular fluid and granulosa cells, although hyperstimulation may still occur following embryo transfer in these IVF patients (29).

## CLINICAL PARAMETERS

Clinical parameters of response to ovarian hyperstimulation may have potential use as adjunctive criteria in assessing follicular maturity. A clinical shift is considered to have occurred when 30% or more of cells of the lateral vaginal wall are pkynotic and at least four of the following characteristics of cervical change are present: mucus volume greater than or equal to 0.2 ml, spinnbarkeit greater than or equal to 10 cc, ferning pattern seen, acellular quality of mucus, dilatation of external cervical os (39). In contrast to the natural menstrual cycle, vaginal cytologic maturation lags behind the rise in peripheral estrogen blood levels. This may be due to a more rapid rise in estrogen production in stimulation cycles. The cytologic changes can be influenced by the patient's prior estrogen status and the presence of an infection (20). The cervical score reflects a rise in estrogen concentration with the initiation of hMG or CC therapy but is unable to distinguish among different elevated estrogen levels. Due to the greater degree of variability inherent in clinical monitoring techniques, these findings are generally not as reliable as laboratory or radiologic criteria. Nevertheless, they may provide additional information on which to base therapy decisions. A clinical shift of 2–3 days prior to cessation of hMG is considered a favorable sign of follicular maturity.

## SPONTANEOUS LH SURGE

In the normal menstrual cycle, a spontaneous midcycle LH surge usually occurs when peripheral estradiol levels reach 200–300 pg/ml; however, when menotropins are administered to stimulate multiple follicular development, spontaneous LH-FSH surges develop in only a minority of patients despite estradiol concentrations in excess of 300 pg/ml for several days (25). Inhibin is secreted in large amounts by the developing follicles when stimulated by exogenous FSH (60). In addition, the preovulatory follicle may secrete another nonsteroidal factor or factors that inhibit the rise in gonadotropins by counter-balancing the positive feedback effect of estradiol on the hypothalamic-pituitary unit (51).

The probability that an LH surge will occur in association with ovarian hyperstimulation is influenced to some extent by the stimulation protocol employed. Although the techniques of monitoring LH do vary, several reports have suggested a higher frequency of spontaneous LH surges in patients treated with hMG only as compared to regimens using both CC and hMG (92). Other studies have refuted this (5). The incidence of this phenomenon ranges from 20–33% in hMG schedules and 9.1–34.0% in CC/hMG protocols (5, 49, 92). Premature luteinization of follicles prior to ovum collection results in impaired fertilization and embryonic development. Hence, identification of an endogenous LH rise in women undergoing controlled ovarian hyperstimulation may advance the time of oocyte retrieval or may be reason for cycle cancellation because of its adverse effect on successful conception.

The average estrogen concentrations and follicular dimensions at the time of an LH surge are not significantly different from those measured in patients who have not developed a spontaneous surge by the time of hCG administration (87). Nevertheless discrepancies exist in the literature. Lejeune and colleagues reported that CC/hMG-stimulated IVF cycles in which a spontaneous LH rise occurred were characterized by lower estradiol levels and smaller follicles than similarly treated cycles where an LH rise did not develop prior to hCG (49). Vargyas and colleagues detected endogenous LH surges in some women when the lead follicle was immature according to sonographic criteria (92). A rapid rate of rise of estradiol rather than an absolute peripheral estrogen concentration appears to be strongly correlated with the onset of the gonadotropin rise (44). Additional clues to the occurrence of an early LH surge may include a rapid enlargement in the follicle and a premature fall in serum estradiol in the latter days of hMG stimulation. Spontaneous LH surge patients are more likely to be older and hyperandrogenic.

The inhibition of the LH surge in menotropin cycles is not necessarily an all-or-none phenomenon. Alteration of the hypothalamic-pituitary response to estradiol by follicular factors may lead to a blunted height of the LH surge, which impairs oocyte nuclear or cytoplasmic maturation (28). Testart and colleagues defined the LH surge as an 80% increase in serum LH relative to the mean level of the previous 4 days (88). Others have defined the LH surge as a serum concentration of greater than 12 mIU/ml (75) or a urinary level exceeding 30 IU/liter (49). The presence of a surge is confirmed by a continued rise in LH concentration and an increase in serum progesterone levels. To improve the accuracy of detection of an endogenous gonadotropin rise, frequent blood or urine sampling must be performed from 1–6 times daily during the latter phase of menotropin stimulation. Ovulation occurs 34–36 hours after the onset of the LH surge, 10–20 hours after LH peaks, and 34–36 hours after the estrogen level peaks (15). Many IVF centers that utilize LH surge cycles administer hCG at the time of recognition of the LH rise (72, 93). Oocyte retrieval is rescheduled to occur 15–25 hours from hCG injection or 24–28 hours from the onset of the endogenous LH surge.

Macnamee and Howles (55) and Lopata (52) reported equivalent pregnancy rates among women who underwent oocyte retrieval following the spontaneous LH surge as compared with control patients who were without a surge. In order to achieve this success, intensive monitoring is necessary, which may include LH measurement every 4 hours when certain sonographic or estradiol criteria are reached. Nevertheless, Lejeune and colleagues reported no pregnancies in 21 retrievals of LH surge patients despite serum LH assay every 4 hours (49). Others have described a marked decrease in oocyte recovery rate in CC/hMG cycles in which the LH surge was associated with a peak estradiol level of more than 1200 pg/ml and the development of less than three follicles 14 mm or greater in diameter (24). Because of the generally diminished pregnancy rates, scheduling difficulties, and monitoring inconvenience, most centers have adopted a policy of cycle cancellation in patients who demonstrate a spontaneous LH surge.

Daily progesterone radioimmunoassay during the preovulatory time period offers additional information for therapy decision making. A rising progesterone concentration in conjunction with a falling estradiol level and lack of an LH surge may signify premature luteinization (43). These cycles are associated with a diminished pregnancy rate. In addition, an early elevation in serum progesterone may signal an impending LH surge and allow administration of hCG concomitant with the onset of the surge (81). An alternative to intensive LH/progesterone monitoring is to eliminate the possibility of an endogenous LH surge by administration of a GnRH agonist concurrent with menotropin stimulation. A significant percentage of cycles are salvaged in this manner.

## hCG ADMINISTRATION

hCG is employed in gonadotropin-stimulated cycles to mimic the natural, mid-cycle LH surge necessary for final follicular maturation. Under the influence of LH, the granulosa cells and oocyte-cumulus complex separate from the follicular wall. The cumulus cells undergo significant changes in shape and orientation, leading to expansion of the cumulus mass. In addition, meiosis proceeds beyond the arrested prophase I stage.

Higher pregnancy rates have been achieved in ovulation induction regimens with the use of hCG as compared to reliance on the endogenous LH rise. Nevertheless, the timing of administration of hCG is critical to the collection of oocytes at the appropriate developmental stage. If hCG is given too late, one or more of the most advanced follicles may yield fragmented, postmature oocytes of low potential embryogenic viability (16). The preovulatory LH/hCG surge may promote atresia of the large antral follicles with LH receptors (13). Conversely, if hCG is injected too early in the induction, the recruited follicles may be intercepted before adequate completion of the maturation process.

The criteria that should be assessed in determining the appropriate timing of hCG administration may include the number and sizes of the lead follicles, estrogen concentration and its rate of rise, length of ovarian stimulation, vaginal cytology and cervical mucus characteristics, and evidence of LH or progesterone rise. Isolated estradiol assays are not a reliable parameter in judging oocyte maturity unless interpreted in context with other data because these values are a reflection of the production by the entire pool of follicles. The rate of rise of estradiol and the duration of the rise have greater diagnostic significance. A plateau or decline in estradiol concentration prior to hCG treatment is associated with a lower pregnancy rate (6). A falling estrogen secretion may be due to premature luteinization or atresia of the lead follicles; conversely, a rapid terminal rise in estradiol may be associated with an imminent LH surge (44). The natural menstrual cycle is characterized by an average of 6 days of continuous estradiol rise prior to the spontaneous LH surge. This apparent optimal length of accelerated follicular development may hold for stimulated cycles as well. Levran and colleagues reported that oocytes obtained from leading follicles in hMG and CC/hMG cycles in which hCG was given after 6 days of estradiol rise had the greatest potential for inducing pregnancies (50). The day of onset of estradiol rise was defined as a minimum increase of 20% over the baseline concentration that continued over the subsequent days of ovarian stimulation.

A lack of consensus exists regarding whether a delay in the administration of hCG following the final hMG dose leads to improved cytoplasmic oocyte maturation and interfollicular synchronization. Jones and colleagues reported a higher pregnancy rate in IVF cycles in which the dosing interval from hMG to hCG was increased to 50–60 hours; however, there was no difference in the fertilization and embryo transfer rates at hMG-hCG time lapses of less than 50 hours (40). Conversely, Laufer and colleagues found that prolongation of this interval beyond 24 hours resulted in a significant increase in the proportion of nonfertilized and degenerated oocytes, possibly due to atretic changes in the lead follicles (46). Ben-Rafael and colleagues have described no significant differences in oocyte recovery, fertilization, and cleavage in patients receiving hCG at intervals of 24, 48, 72, and 96 hours after the last hMG dose; nevertheless, delay in hCG administration by 72 and 96 hours resulted in an increased percentage of cancelled cycles due to a sharp drop in estradiol (6). The specific criteria that favor a dosing interval less than approximately 36 hours include a plateau in estradiol levels from the previous day, a lead follicle greater than 1.8 cm in diameter, and a history of a spontaneous LH surge in a previous ovarian stimulation cycle.

Doses of hCG ranging from 2000 to 10,000 IU have been used by IVF programs to induce final follicular maturation. Five thousand or ten thousand IU are recommended due to a significantly lower successful oocyte recovery rate with 2000 IU doses of hCG (1). The lower doses may cause an incomplete maturation of the cumulus-oocyte complex.

## Methods of Controlled Ovarian Hyperstimulation

In 1981, Trounson and colleagues reported the development of intrauterine pregnancies through multiple embryo transfer in CC-stimulated IVF cycles (90). Since then, various combinations of gonadotropins, CC, and GnRH agonists have been utilized for follicular stimulation in an effort to obtain the maximum number of fertilizable oocytes without disrupting luteal phase endometrial morphology. These protocols will be briefly reviewed.

### Clomiphene Citrate

Regimens of CC alone and in combination with hCG as a substitute for the midcycle LH surge were proposed as a method by which more than one dominant follicle could be recruited. CC 50–150 mg has been introduced on day 5 of the spontaneous cycle and continued for 5 consecutive days. Due to the great variability of follicular response and a 30–50% frequency of spontaneous LH surges prior to hCG administration in patients stimulated by CC, other protocols have been pursued (40). Experiments performed in animal models have revealed that the critical time period for recruitment and selection of the dominant follicle lies in the early follicular phase of the primate menstrual cycle. In order to promote growth and avert follicular atresia, clinical trials of CC were altered to commence on cycle day 2 or 3 (57). Multiple follicles were stimulated; however, inadequate continuous gonadotropin support resulted in an overall decline in the collection of mature oocytes. The combination CC/hMG regimen was devised to overcome this deficiency.

### CC/hMG

Reports from several IVF centers have generally indicated that an improved rate of oocyte collection, cleavage, and embryo transfer is achieved via CC/hMG protocols as compared to reliance on CC stimulation alone; nevertheless, the differences in ongoing pregnancy rates among the various treatments are less marked. Yee and Vargas, utilizing a regimen of CC 100 mg/day on days 3–7 concurrent with one ampule per day of hMG, described a 19% pregnancy rate per laparoscopic retrieval; this compared to their CC stimulation success rate of 11% (96). Conversely, although Diamond and colleagues obtained a statistically significant increase in total numbers of developing follicles, oocytes recovered, and embryos replaced by administering CC 50–100 mg on cycle days 3–7 and hMG two ampules per day beginning on cycle day 6 or 7, they found no difference in pregnancy rates between this schedule and single-agent therapy with CC or hMG (21). More recently, Pampiglione and colleagues reported a pregnancy rate per embryo transfer of 30.2% after treating patients with CC 100 mg from days 2–6 and hMG two to three ampules daily from day 4 onward (69). Continued trials of such combination regimens have suggested their general superiority over sole CC stimulation. CC is the first of the two agents administered in the majority of these combination schedules; hMG dosage may overlap or follow CC treatment and may be given daily or at less frequent time intervals. Mature follicles derived from this mode of therapy exhibit similar sonographic dimensions to preovulatory follicles in the unstimulated menstrual cycle.

### Gonadotropins

IVF protocols that include only gonadotropins as the stimulus for follicular development were devised to avoid any potential deleterious effect that CC might have on the ovary or endometrium. CC may be an estrogen agonist or an antagonist depending on the hormonal environment at its site of action. Previous reports have suggested that a high incidence of luteal phase defects exists in normally cycling patients who have received CC (17). This disorder may be due to a competitive inhibition of estrogen receptors in the endometrium or, more likely, a direct antiestrogen action of CC on ovarian steroidogenesis. The ovum fertilized in vitro enters the uterine cavity approximately 2 days earlier than it would if fertilization occurred in vivo; hence, a delay in endometrial maturation may be particularly detrimental to embryonic implantation. Some degree of corpus luteum insufficiency also may be present in hMG-stimulated IVF cycles; however, a recent study of endometrial biopsies taken on the second day after follicular aspiration revealed a significantly higher rate of normal luteal phase histology in hMG/hCG recipients than in patients treated with CC/hCG or CC/hMG/hCG (86).

The original two-cell theory for estradiol production proposed an equivalent importance of FSH and LH. LH stimulates androstenedione secretion by the theca cell; these weak androgens are aromatized to form estradiol by the FSH-sensitive granulosa cell. Reflecting this theory of gonadotropin action, urinary menotropin preparations were originally prepared at an empiric 1:1 ratio of FSH to LH (37). One ampule of Pergonal contains the equivalent of 75 IU of FSH and 75 IU of LH in the form of a lyophilized powder, which is reconstituted with normal saline for intramuscular injection.

The timing of initiation of gonadotropin therapy for controlled ovarian hyperstimulation in normally cycling women is critical for achieving optimal folliculogenesis. Beginning treatment in the luteal phase of the antecedent menstrual cycle may prolong corpus luteum function, stimulate progesterone secretion, and lead to inadequate development and poor receptiveness of the endometrium (82); however if hMG administration is delayed beyond selection of the dominant follicle, the remaining follicles in the cohort would already have begun the process of atresia and consequently have significantly compromised developmental potential. Institution of therapy on cycle day 3 generally provides favorable follicular recruitment. This supraphysiologic exogenous gonadotropin stimulation is temporarily correlated with the perimenstrual rise in serum FSH that occurs in the spontaneous cycle.

Sensitivity to menotropins varies among individuals. A direct relationship exists between the patient's weight and her hMG requirements. Women who are not obese are likely to respond to lower doses of hMG than patients who are greater than 10% and particularly greater than 25% of their ideal body weight (14). In addition, individuals with severe hypothalamic chronic anovulation syndrome generally require a larger than average number of ampules of hMG per cycle to achieve adequate folliculogenesis. Presumably, more FSH is needed to induce estradiol production and up-regulation of granulosa cell FSH receptors in chronic hypoestrogenic conditions. Conversely, patients with high basal LH-FSH levels as found in polycystic ovarian disease may benefit from lower daily doses of hMG due to a more favorable hormonal milieu at the ovarian and uterine levels. In the average estrogenic patient, a maintenance dose of two ampules of hMG per day appears optimal for oocyte development. Higher hMG doses may lead to a greater percentage of atretic follicles and premature ovulations (7). In addition, very high estradiol levels derived through marked ovarian stimulation may yield an endometrial environment hostile to nidation (7).

Further alterations in stimulation protocols have attempted to enhance FSH recruitment of follicles from the gonadotropin-sensitive pool by imitating the usual early follicular phase rise of FSH in the spontaneous menstrual cycle without exposing the follicles to high concentrations of LH. The FSH contained within the hMG mixture is the strongly dominant component in stimulating folliculogenesis. In vitro studies suggest that the LH in hMG may impair oocyte development and successful implantation by altering theca androgen metabolism (71). Exposure of the ovaries to a high level of LH during the first half of the follicular phase may be particularly detrimental to IVF success (53). In an effort to counterbalance these potentially conflicting gonadotropin effects during ovulation induction, additional stimulation in the form of purified urinary FSH (hFSH, Metrodin) has been included in the critical first 2–3 days of therapy (10). This preparation contains 75 IU FSH activity and less than 1 IU LH activity per ampule. Although this modification of the protocol offers theoretic advantages (1), the published reports have not consistently shown an improved pregnancy rate (9). Moreover, follicular stimulation with hFSH alone appears to offer no definite enhancement of oocyte quality or viable gestation rate (48).

## PROGRAMMED CYCLES WITH ORAL CONTRACEPTIVES

Synthetic steroids have been employed to regulate menses as part of fixed ovulation induction protocols (27). These programmed cycles may increase the efficiency of an IVF center by enabling an advanced scheduling of oocyte retrieval and permitting a synchronization of patient entry into active ovarian stimulation at any given time. Progestins and combination oral contraceptive agents act centrally on the hypothalamus and pituitary and locally on the ovary to inhibit the normal selection process that occurs in early follicular development. Suppression of luteal phase FSH secretion by these steroids may create a more homogenous cohort of follicles on initiation of induction (89). In addition, studies have suggested a lower incidence of spontaneous LH surges in patients pretreated with norethindrone 2.5–10.0 mg/day or low-dose oral contraceptives (89). Ovulation induction is generally begun 3 days after withdrawal of the steroids. Nevertheless, disadvantages do exist with this form of therapy. The ovary remains insensitive to gonadotropin stimulation in direct proportion to the time interval of steroid suppression. This prolongation of the latent phase of follicular development is more pronounced with contraceptive pill administration for more than 30 days (57). Fewer preovulatory follicles are obtained after pretreatment, and the cycle cancellation rate may be higher due to inadequate ovarian response to stimulation. Several reports have indicated that pregnancy rates from these IVF cycles are equivalent to nonprogrammed cycles in patients who have embryos transferred (27, 59, 89). Due to the drawbacks described above, GnRH analogs are the preferred agents for cycle regulation in IVF protocols.

## COMBINED GnRH ANALOG/hMG THERAPY

Hypothalamic-pituitary functions contribute substantially to the variability of ovarian response during gonadotropin treatment. Clinical trials of menotropin stimulation in anovulatory patients have revealed a significantly higher conception rate per cycle and a lower spontaneous abortion rate in patients with hypogonadotropic hypogonadism as compared to other conditions such as polycystic ovarian disease (97). This recognition has promoted interest in the induction of a reversible hypogonadotropic state in women undergoing controlled ovarian hyperstimulation for IVF. Initial creation of a pharmacologic hypophysectomy should provide a more synchronous follicular cohort, diminish the variability in response between patients, and minimize the occurrence of adverse events such as premature luteinization or early ovulation.

Suppression of endogenous gonadotropin secretion may be achieved by prolonged administration of a GnRH agonist. Currently, leuprolide acetate (Lupron) is the only agonist available for clinical use in the United States, although many other formulations are employed elsewhere. These hypothalamic peptide analogs have a high affinity to the GnRH receptor and a decreased resistance to degeneration as compared to native releasing hormone. Initial exposure of the pituitary gonadotrope cells to the agonist results in a prompt stimulation of LH and FSH release. The circulatory levels of gonadotropins will peak 4–6 hours after GnRH agonist administration at concentrations several times those present during the spontaneous midcycle surge of these hormones (75). The LH and FSH will remain elevated in the peripheral blood for approximately 10 hours (54).

In response to the rise in gonadotropin secretion, serum estradiol levels will increase to a peak of 2–4 times the base levels at 7–16 hours after analog

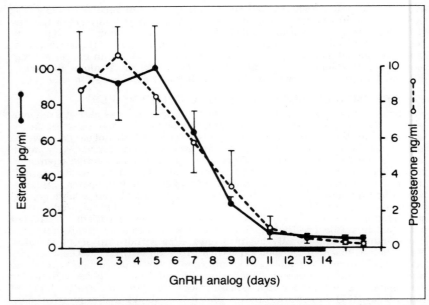

**Fig. 8-6.** Estradiol and progesterone levels (mean ± SEM) immediately prior to and following initiation of GnRH analog treatment during the midluteal phase of the menstrual cycle. (From D. de Ziegler et al. Suppression of the ovary using a gonadotropin releasing-hormone agonist prior to stimulation for oocyte retrieval. *Fertil. Steril.* 48:807, 1987. With permission.)

injection (54). Repeat exposure of the pituitary gland to GnRH agonists results in a reduction of available GnRH receptors, an impairment of postreceptor mechanisms, and ultimately an unresponsiveness of the gonadotrope to GnRH. Basal and pulsatile secretion of FSH and LH are diminished. Estrogen levels decline due to a lack of follicular stimulation.

The rapidity of endogenous gonadotropin suppression depends on the stage of the menstrual cycle in which the GnRH agonist is introduced. A significantly more prompt and consistent inhibition of follicular activity is noted when the medication is begun in the midluteal time period as compared to the follicular phase (61). With luteal phase initiation, corpus luteal steroidogenesis is stimulated, and menses may be delayed up to 6 days beyond the expected time of onset. Progesterone production rises for approximately 3 days before declining to basal levels after 5–11 days of therapy (18). (Fig. 8-6). The early elevation in progesterone concentration presumably leads to a blunting of response of the pituitary gonadotropes to endogenous releasing hormone (2). Conversely, if GnRH agonist therapy is instituted in the follicular phase, the initial rise in FSH and LH secretion can stimulate the further development of a cohort of follicles, resulting in elevations in estradiol for up to 3 weeks.

GnRH analog administration inhibits the early developmental asynchrony of follicles that occurs in the late luteal phase of natural cycles in response to increased secretion of FSH. As a result, menotropin stimulation following GnRH analog pretreatment generally yields a higher number of preovulatory follicles for IVF (23). Variability in response among patients and for an individual patient from one cycle to the next is diminished in most cases. Although the immunoreactive LH concentration remains unchanged, prolonged GnRH analog therapy suppresses circulating levels of bioactive LH, thereby preventing premature luteinization. An early rise in progesterone secretion by the luteinized follicle prior to ovulation may adversely affect oocyte quality and endometrial maturation. With decreased incidence of the spontaneous LH surge, the cycle cancellation rate due to poor response to stimulation falls to approximately 7% (23, 62). In addition, the decline in bioactive LH results in a decline in ovarian androgen production and an improved follicular environment for oocyte maturation. Patients with an elevated baseline day 3 LH-FSH ratio prior to initiation of GnRH analog therapy are particularly benefitted by such treatment; oocyte fertilization and pregnancy rates are increased, and the spontaneous abortion rate is decreased as compared to cycles in which hMG alone is used (23). The enhanced efficacy of combination GnRH analog/hMG stimulation regimens is not as uniform in those patients who have previously responded poorly to hMG therapy alone. Women who are generally least benefitted are those who have an elevated basal FSH level, a finding suggestive of diminished ovarian reserve.

Patients require significantly more exogenous gonadotropin stimulation in leuprolide/hMG cycles to achieve a desired logarithmic rise in circulating estradiol. As much as 3 times the total quantity of hMG is required in GnRH analog/hMG cycles as compared to CC/hMG cycles (34). Moreover, 2–3 additional days of stimulation are often necessary for adequate follicular development (23); presumably, this prolongation is due to an absence of responsive follicles at the onset of hMG therapy. Leuprolide has no measurable effect on human fertilization, cleavage, or embryo growth rate. Serum, follicular, and peritoneal fluid concentrations of leuprolide are undetectable 2 days after discontinuation of the medication, well before the time of embryo transfer (22).

An alternative technique in follicular stimulation takes advantage of the initial flare in pituitary gonadotropin secretion by introducing the GnRH analog on cycle day 1 or 2 (77). Serum FSH values become elevated 1.5–6.0-fold over baseline to peak on day 3 of agonist administration. Menotropin therapy is usually initiated on cycle day 2 or 3. By continuing the GnRH analog treatment, endogenous gonadotropin secretion is suppressed to near basal levels by the late follicular phase of stimulation, thereby inhibiting premature luteinization. Potential advantages of this short-term protocol included lowered cost and duration of treatment; however, markedly elevated serum LH concentrations during the agonistic phase of analog action stimulate progesterone production by the ovary (Fig. 8-7). Reported success rates using this short-term combined protocol have been variable. Although some centers have achieved excellent results (77), others have described oocyte atresia and reduced embryo quality as compared with stimulation cycles that were pretreated with GnRH analog (12, 53). A marked rise in LH and progesterone secretion during early follicular development may permanently impair oocyte maturation.

The current John Hopkins Hospital IVF Center protocol for all patients who have not previously undergone ovarian stimulation includes pituitary suppression with leuprolide acetate followed by menotropin therapy. Leuprolide 1 mg SC is introduced on cycle day 20 of the antecedent menstrual cycle and is continued daily until the Friday or Saturday following the onset of menses. On that day, baseline sonographic and estrogen studies are obtained to assess the adequacy of ovarian suppression. If the estradiol concentration is less than 12 pg/ml and if no follicle is greater than 1.0 cm in diameter, the leuprolide dose is decreased to 0.5 mg SC per day and menotropin stimulation is initiated. If these criteria are not met, the GnRH agonist is continued at the dosage of 1 mg/day for an additional 3–7 days. The average length of menotropin stimulation prior to hCG administration in our program is 9–11 days; by introducing therapy on a Friday or Saturday, the oocyte retrievals are more likely to occur during midweek. Continuation of the leuprolide until the day of hCG injection maintains pituitary suppression and prevents premature luteinization. Decreasing the daily dosage of leuprolide to 0.5 mg provides adequate pituitary inhibition

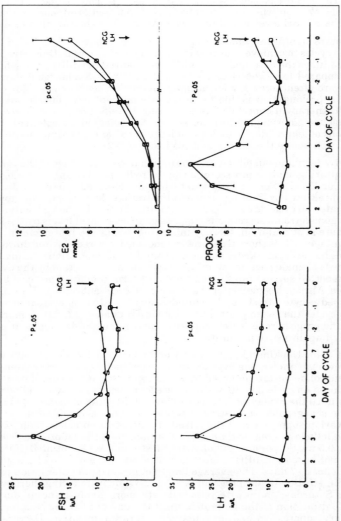

Fig. 8-7. Serum levels of FSH, LH, estradiol ($E_2$), and progesterone (mean ± SEM) in subjects treated with hMG (△) and leuprolide acetate/hMG (□). Both leuprolide and hMG were initiated on cycle day 2. Late follicular concentrations were normalized to the day of hCG or the onset of the LH surge. Note early "flare" in LH, progesterone, and FSH values with concurrent introduction of GnRH analog and hMG. (From M. Sathanandan et al. Adjuvant leuprolide in normal, abnormal, and poor responders to controlled ovarian hyperstimulation for in vitro fertilization/gamete intrafallopian transfer. *Fertil. Steril.* 51:998, 1989. With permission.)

Table 8-1. Outcome per stage of therapy

| | |
|---|---|
| Successful ovulation induction | 93–95% |
| Successful oocyte retrieval | 88–89% |
| Fertilization rate | 79–82% |
| Pregnancy rate per embryo transfer | 23% |
| Cycle cancellation due to poor stimulation | 5–7% |
| Premature ovulation | 1–2% |

during the stimulation phase but does not significantly affect ovarian steroidogenesis as has been reported with higher doses of the analog (4).

Our patients receive two ampules of hFSH and two ampules of hMG at 4 P.M. on the first day of stimulation. On the second day of stimulation, two ampules of hFSH at 8 A.M. and two ampules of hMG at 4 P.M. are administered. Two ampules of hFSH are administered at 4 P.M. on cycle days 3 and 4. Additional hMG (one to two ampules) may be given on cycle days 3 and 4, depending on patient estradiol response. Adjustment of the above dosages are made if the patient weighs less than 55 kg due to the decreased gonadotropin requirements of these women (32). The treatment is individualized thereafter based on follicular response as assessed by daily morning estradiol assays and sonographic and clinical examinations. Two ampules of hMG are given per day following cycle day 4 unless this dosage is insufficient to maintain an exponential rise of estradiol or an approximate 2-mm daily growth in the diameter of the dominant follicles. If the hMG dose is three ampules or less, the medication is received as a single afternoon injection. If four or more ampules are required, the dosage is divided as per the schedule on days 1–4 of stimulation. hCG is administered between 30–36 hours after the final dose of hMG when at least two follicles average 1.8 cm in diameter. Serum LH and progesterone are not routinely measured. The oocyte retrieval is performed 34–36 hours after the hCG injection. Cycle cancellation is considered if a plateauing of estradiol concentration occurs for 3 consecutive days or estradiol declines over 2 consecutive days despite increasing doses of hMG. In addition, if less than three codominant follicles develop during the induction process, there is diminished likelihood of collecting an optimal number of preovulatory oocytes. Use of this follicular stimulation protocol at the Johns Hopkins Hospital during the first 6 months of 1989 yielded the statistics for each phase of therapy listed in Table 8-1.

## OVARIAN HYPERSTIMULATION SYNDROME

Ovarian hyperstimulation syndrome is the most serious complication of gonadotropin therapy. The varying presentations of this syndrome arise 5–8 days after hCG injection due to marked ovarian enlargement and increased vascular permeability. Three clinical categories of involvement have been established based on the severity of symptoms (20). Patients with mild hyperstimulation experience lower abdominal discomfort and ovarian enlargement up to 5 × 5 cm. Moderate hyperstimulation is characterized by greater abdominal pain, ascitic abdominal distention, and ovarian enlargement up to 12 × 12 cm. Third-space fluid sequestration due to increased capillary extravasation may lead to weight gain of up to 10 pounds. With severe hyperstimulation, the ovaries are palpable abdominally, and additional findings may include ascites, hydrothorax, pericardial effusion, oliguria, hemoconcentration, hypercoagulation, and electrolyte and liver enzyme abnormalities (79).

The incidence of ovarian hyperstimulation syndrome ranges from 3–83% for the mild forms and from 0.4–4.0% for the more severe categories (66). The milder variant is a common and acceptable development in women undergoing induction of multiple follicular maturation for IVF; however, the more severe forms bear significant morbidity. Several factors have been identified as predictive for

**Table 8-2. Factors predictive for the development of ovarian hyperstimulation syndrome**

Young age
Lean body weight
Chronic anovulation with elevated LH-FSH ratio
Very high preovulatory levels of estrogen
Dyssynchrony of recruitment with multiple small follicles present on the day of
  hCG

the development of ovarian hyperstimulation syndrome (Table 8-2). Young, thin, hyperandrogenic women exhibit an increased ovarian sensitivity to exogenous gonadotropin therapy as compared with patients not developing complications of hyperstimulation (66). Small follicles with a mean diameter of 7.5 mm continue to grow after hCG administration, thereby increasing estrogen production and contributing to the cascade of events that compose the hyperstimulation syndrome (11). Severe fluid shifts have been caused by follicular stimulation with hMG or hFSH alone as well as in conjunction with CC or GnRH analog therapy; however, hCG administration is mandatory for the development of the syndrome.

The pathophysiologic mechanisms responsible for ovarian hyperstimulation syndrome have not been fully delineated. Massive ovarian enlargement due to the development of multiple follicular and corpus luteum cysts and an increased capillary permeability have been linked to ovarian angiogenesis and activation of the renin-angiotensin cascade (65). Histamine and prostaglandins have been implicated as factors promoting altered vascular membrane permeability (78).

Treatment is tailored to achieve symptomatic relief. Mild to moderate conditions require outpatient observation and restriction of activities. Women with severe hyperstimulation require hospitalization and frequent monitoring of vital signs, urine output, blood electrolytes, and coagulation parameters. Plasma expanders may be necessary to increase intravascular colloid osmotic pressure. Renal dialysis and ventilatory support are rarely required. Ovarian rupture and torsion are additional very infrequent complications; oophorectomy is usually unavoidable in such instances. The patient should begin to diurese within 3–7 days after menstruation if she is not pregnant. If conception occurs, a slow improvement in hyperstimulation symptoms occurs over 6–8 weeks.

## LUTEAL PHASE SUPPORT

Elevated estradiol secretion arising from multiple follicular stimulation has a detrimental effect on successful embryo implantation in IVF patients (26). Several studies have confirmed the existence of a shortened luteal phase and decreased progesterone production as reflected by urinary pregnanediol levels in gonadotropin-stimulated cycles (63, 73). High luteal phase estrogen production may inhibit pituitary gonadotropin secretion and disrupt corpus luteal function (58). Patients who receive combination GnRH analog/hMG therapy may be even more predisposed to develop luteal phase insufficiency due to the analog's inhibition of endogenous LH secretion; nevertheless, the efficacy of progesterone support in the luteal phase following IVF-embryo transfer has not been conclusively demonstrated (56). In order to promote an improved endometrial environment for nidation following ovarian stimulation via the above protocol, we supplement the luteal phase with progesterone-in-oil 25 mg IM every 12 hours beginning the evening before the embryo transfer. In addition, hCG 5000 IU is administered 4 days after follicular puncture to stimulate endogenous progesterone production. A quantitative hCG titer is obtained on all patients 12 days after embryo transfer. If positive, the intramuscular injections are discontinued, and the patient begins therapy with 25-mg progesterone vaginal suppositories every 12 hours. These are administered through the first trimester of pregnancy. A very low spontaneous abortion rate has been achieved using the above treatment protocols.

## REFERENCES

1. Abdalla, H. I., et al. The effect of the dose of human chorionic gonadotropin and the type of gonadotropin stimulation on oocyte recovery rates in an in vitro fertilization program. *Fertil. Steril.* 48, 958, 1987.
2. Araki, S., et al. Reduction in pituitary desensitization and prolongation of gonadotropin release by estrogen during continuous administration of gonadotropin-releasing hormone in women: Its antagonism by progesterone. *J. Clin. Endocrinol. Metab.* 60:590, 1985.
3. Baird, D. T. A model for follicular selection and ovulation: Lessons from superovulation. *J. Steroid Biochem.* 27:15, 1987.
4. Barnes, R. B., Scommegna, A., and Schreiber, J. F. Decreased ovarian response to human menopausal gonadotropin caused by subcutaneously administered gonadotropin-releasing hormone agonist. *Fertil. Steril.* 47:512, 1987.
5. Bayly, C. M., McBain, J. C., and Clarke, G. A. Ovarian stimulation regimens in an in vitro fertilization program: A comparative analysis. *Ann. N.Y. Acad. Sci.* 442:123, 1985.
6. Ben-Rafael, Z., et al. Follicular maturation parameters associated with the failure of oocyte retrieval, fertilization, and cleavage in vitro. *Fertil. Steril.* 45:51, 1986.
7. Ben-Rafael, Z., et al. Dose of human menopausal gonadotropin influences the outcome of an in vitro fertilization program. *Fertil. Steril.* 48:964, 1987.
8. Benadiva, C. A., et al. Ovarian response of individuals to different doses of human menopausal gonadotropin. *Fertil. Steril.* 49:997, 1988.
9. Benadiva, C. A., et al. An increased initial follicle-stimulatory hormone/luteinizing hormone ratio does not affect ovarian responses and the outcome of in vitro fertilization. *Fertil. Steril.* 50:777, 1988.
10. Bernardus, R. E., et al. The significance of the ratio of follicle-stimulating hormone and luteinizing hormone in induction of multiple follicular growth. *Fertil. Steril.* 43:373, 1985.
11. Blankstein, J., et al. Ovarian hyperstimulation syndrome: Prediction of number and size of preovulatory ovarian follicles. *Fertil. Steril.* 47:597, 1987.
12. Brzyski, R. G., et al. Follicular atresia associated with concurrent initiation of gonadotropin-releasing hormone agonist and follicle-stimulating hormone for oocyte recruitment. *Fertil. Steril.* 50:917, 1988.
13. Chikazawa, K., Araki, S., and Tamada, T. Morphological and endocrinological studies on follicular development during the human menstrual cycle. *J. Clin. Endocrinol. Metab.* 62:305, 1986.
14. Chong, A. P., Rafael, R. W., and Forte, C. C. Influence of weight in the induction of ovulation with human menopausal gonadotropin and human chorionic gonadotropin. *Fertil. Steril.* 46:599, 1986.
15. Collins, W. P., et al. The concentrations of urinary oestrone-3-glucuronide, LH, and pregnanediol-3 α-glucuronide as indices of ovarian function. *Acta Endocrinol.* 90:336, 1979.
16. Collins, R., Williams, R. F., and Hodgen, G. D. Endocrine consequences of prolonged ovarian hyperstimulation: Hyperprolactinemia, follicular atresia, and premature luteinization. *Fertil. Steril.* 40:436, 1984.
17. Cook, C. L., et al. Induction of luteal phase defect with clomiphene citrate. *Am. J. Obstet. Gynecol.* 149:613, 1984.
18. de Ziegler, D., et al. Suppression of the ovary using a gonadotropin releasing-hormone agonist prior to stimulation for oocyte retrieval. *Fertil. Steril.* 48:807, 1987.
19. DeCherney, A. H., and Laufer, N. The monitoring of ovulation induction using ultrasound and estrogen. *Clin. Obstet. Gynecol.* 27:993, 1984.
20. Diamond, M. P., and Wentz, A. C. Ovulation induction with human menopausal gonadotropins. *Obstet. Gynecol. Surv.* 41:480, 1986.

21. Diamond, M. P., et al. Comparison of human menopausal gonadotropin, clomiphene citrate, and combined human menopausal gonadotropin-clomiphene citrate stimulation protocols for in vitro fertilization. *Fertil. Steril.* 46:1108, 1986.

22. Dodson, W. C., et al. Leuprolide acetate: Serum and follicular fluid concentrations and effects on human fertilization, embryo growth, and granulosa-lutein cell progesterone accumulation in vitro. *Fertil. Steril.* 50:612, 1988.

23. Droesch, K., et al. Value of suppression with a gonadotropin-releasing hormone agonist prior to gonadotropin stimulation for in vitro fertilization. *Fertil. Steril.* 51:292, 1989.

24. Eibschitz, I., Belaisch-Ailart, J. C., and Frydman, R. In vitro fertilization management and results in stimulated cycles with spontaneous luteinizing hormone discharge. *Fertil. Steril.* 45:231, 1986.

25. Ferraretti, A. P., et al. Serum luteinizing hormone during ovulation induction with human menopausal gonadotropin for in vitro fertilization in normally menstruating women. *Fertil. Steril.* 40:742, 1983.

26. Forman, R., et al. Evidence for an adverse effect of elevated serum estradiol concentrations on embryo implantation. *Fertil. Steril.* 49:118, 1988.

27. Frydman, R., et al. A new approach to follicular stimulation for in vitro fertilization; programmed oocyte retrieval. *Fertil. Steril.* 46:657, 1986.

28. Glasier, A., et al. Superovulation with exogenous gonadotropins does not inhibit the luteinizing hormone surge. *Fertil. Steril.* 49:81, 1988.

29. Golan, A., et al. Ovarian hyperstimulation syndrome following D-Trp-6-luteinizing hormone-releasing hormone microcapsules and menotropin for in vitro fertilization. *Fertil. Steril.* 50:912, 1988.

30. Gourgeon, A. Dynamics of follicular growth: A model from preliminary results. *Hum. Reprod.* 1:81, 1986.

31. Hackeloer, B-J., and Sallam, H. N. Ultrasound scanning of ovarian follicles. *Clin. Obstet. Gynecol.* 10:603, 1983.

32. Halme, J., et al. Lower doses of human menopausal gonadotropin are associated with improved success with in vitro fertilization in women with low body weight. *Am. J. Obstet. Gynecol.* 158:64, 1988.

33. Hodgen, G. D. The dominant ovarian follicle. *Fertil. Steril.* 38:281, 1982.

34. Horvath, P. M., et al. Exogenous gonadotropin requirements are increased in leuprolide suppressed women undergoing ovarian stimulation. *Fertil. Steril.* 49:159, 1988.

35. Hull, M. E., et al. Correlation of serum estradiol levels and ultrasound monitoring to assess follicular maturation. *Fertil. Steril.* 46:42, 1986.

36. Insler, V., and Potashnik, G. Monitoring of follicular development in gonadotropin-stimulated cycles. In H. Beier and H. R. Lindner (eds.), *Fertilization of the Human Egg In Vitro: Biologic Basis and Applications.* Berlin: Springer-Verlag, 1983. P. 111.

37. Jacobson, A., and Marshall, J. R. Ovulatory response rate with human menopausal gonadotropins of varying FSH/LH ratios. *Fertil. Steril.* 20:171, 1969.

38. Jones, G. S. Update on in vitro fertilization. *Endocr. Rev.* 5:62, 1984.

39. Jones, H. W., Jr., et al. The program for in vitro fertilization at Norfolk. *Fertil. Steril.* 38:14, 1982.

40. Jones, H. W., Jr., et al. The importance of the follicular phase to success and failure in in vitro fertilization. *Fertil. Steril.* 40:317, 1983.

41. Kerin, J. F., et al. Morphological and functional relations of Graafian follicle growth to ovulation in women using ultrasonic, laparoscopic and biochemical measurements. *Br. J. Obstet. Gynaecol.* 88:81, 1981.

42. Kerin, J. F., et al. The effect of Clomid induced superovulation on human follicular and luteal function for extracorporeal fertilization and embryo transfer. *Clin. Reprod. Fertil.* 2:129, 1983.

43. Kerin, J. F., et al. Endocrinology of ovarian stimulation for in vitro fertilization. *Aust. N. Z. J. Obstet Gynaecol.* 24:121, 1984.

44. Kreiner, D., et al. Spontaneous luteinizing hormone (LH) surges are associated

with more rapidly increasing estradiol ($E_2$) and follicle stimulating hormone (FSH) in in vitro fertilization and embryo transfer. *J. In Vitro Fert. Embryo Transf.* 5:265, 1988.

45. Laufer, N., et al. The use of high dose human menopausal gonadotropin in an in vitro fertilization program. *Fertil. Steril.* 40:734, 1983.

46. Laufer, N., et al. Delaying human chorionic gonadotropin administration in human menopausal gonadotropin-induced cycles decreases successful in vitro fertilization of human oocytes. *Fertil. Steril.* 42:198, 1984.

47. Laufer, N., et al. The association between preovulatory serum 17 β estradiol pattern and conception in human menopausal gonadotropin–human chorionic gonadotropin stimulation. *Fertil. Steril.* 46:73, 1986.

48. Lavy, G., et al. Ovarian stimulation for in vitro fertilization and embryo transfer, human menopausal gonadotropin versus pure human follicle stimulating hormone: a randomized prospective study. *Fertil. Steril.* 50:74, 1988.

49. Lejeune, B., et al. In vitro fertilization and embryo transfer as related to endogenous luteinizing hormone rise or human chorionic gonadotropin administration. *Fertil. Steril.* 45:377, 1986.

50. Levran, D., et al. Analysis of outcome of in vitro fertilization in relation to the timing of human chorionic gonadotropin administration by the duration of estradiol rise in stimulated cycles. *Fertil. Steril.* 44:335, 1985.

51. Littman, B. A., and Hodgen, G. D. Human menopausal gonadotropin stimulation in monkeys: Blockade of the luteinizing hormone surge by a highly transient ovarian factor. *Fertil. Steril.* 41:440, 1984.

52. Lopata, A. Concepts in human in vitro fertilization and embryo transfer. *Fertil. Steril.* 40:289, 1983.

53. Loumaye, E., et al. Hormonal changes induced by short-term administration of a gonadotropin-releasing hormone agonist during ovarian hyperstimulation for in vitro fertilization and their consequences for embryo development. *Fertil. Steril.* 51:105, 1989.

54. MacLachlan, V., et al. Luteinizing-hormone-releasing hormone agonist treatment in patients with previously failed folliculogenesis during in vitro fertilization therapy. *N.Y. Acad. Sci.* 541:60, 1988.

55. Macnamee, M. D., and Howles, C. M. The occurrence, characteristics, and management of the LH surge in IVF. *Hum. Reprod.* 2(Suppl. 1):46, 1987.

56. Macnamee, M. D., Edwards, R. G., and Howles, C. M. The influence of stimulation regimes and luteal phase support on the outcome of IVF. *Hum. Reprod.* 3(Suppl. 2):43, 1988.

57. Marrs, R. P., et al. The effect of the time of initiation of clomiphene citrate on multiple follicular development for human in vitro fertilization and embryo replacement procedures. *Fertil. Steril.* 41:682, 1984.

58. Martikainen, H., et al. Anterior pituitary dysfunction during the luteal phase following ovarian hyperstimulation. *Fertil. Steril.* 47:446, 1987.

59. Mashiach, S., Dor, J., and Goldenberg, M. Protocols for induction of ovulation: The concept of programmed cycles. *Ann. N.Y. Acad. Sci.* 541:37, 1988.

60. McLachlan, R. I., et al. Plasma inhibin levels during gonadotropin-induced ovarian hyperstimulation for IVF: A new index of follicular function? *Lancet* 1:1233, 1986.

61. Meldrum, D. R., et al. Timing of initiation and dose schedule of leuprolide influence the time course of ovarian suppression. *Fertil. Steril.* 50:400, 1988.

62. Meldrum, D. R., et al. Routine ovarian stimulation for oocyte retrieval. *Fertil. Steril.* 51:455, 1989.

63. Messinis, I. E., Templeton, A., and Baird, D. T. Luteal phase after ovarian hyperstimulation. *Br. J. Obstet. Gynaecol.* 94:345, 1987.

64. Muasher, S. J., et al. The value of basal and/or stimulated serum gonadotropin levels in prediction of stimulation response and in vitro fertilization outcome. *Fertil. Steril.* 50:298, 1988.

65. Navot, D., et al. Direct correlation between plasma renin activity and severity of the ovarian hyperstimulation syndrome. *Fertil. Steril.* 48:57, 1987.

66. Navot, D., et al. Risk factors and prognostic variables in the ovarian hyperstimulation syndrome. *Am. J. Obstet. Gynecol.* 159:210, 1988.
67. Nayudu, P. L., et al. Follicular characteristics associated with viable pregnancy after in vitro fertilization in humans. *Gamete Res.* 18:37, 1987.
68. Nayudu, P. L., et al. Prediction of outcome in human in vitro fertilization based on follicular and stimulation response variables. *Fertil. Steril.* 51:117, 1989.
69. Pampiglione, J. S., et al. The effect of cycle length on the outcome of in vitro fertilization. *Fertil. Steril.* 50:603, 1988.
70. Pellicer, A., Polan, M. L., and DeCherney, A. H. Improved oocyte quality through improved ovulation induction regimen. *Ann. N.Y. Acad. Sci.* 541:46, 1988.
71. Polan, M. L., Ovulation induction with human menopausal gonadotropin compared to human urinary follicle-stimulating hormone results in a significant shift in follicular fluid androgen levels without discernible differences in granulosa-luteal cell function. *J. Clin. Endocrinol. Metab.* 63:1284, 1986.
72. Punnonen, R., et al. Spontaneous luteinizing hormone surge and cleavage of in vitro fertilized embryos. *Fertil. Steril.* 49:479, 1988.
73. Quigley, M. M. Selection of agents for enhanced follicular recruitment in an in vitro fertilization and embryo replacement program. *Ann. N.Y. Acad. Sci.* 442:96, 1985.
74. Richards, J. S. Maturation of ovarian follicles: actions and interactions of pituitary and ovarian hormones on follicular cell differentiation. *Physiol. Rev.* 60:51, 1980.
75. Rojas, F. J., et al. Assessment of serum luteinizing hormone during ovarian stimulation with gonadotropins. *Hum. Reprod.* 3:207, 1988.
76. Rossavik, I. K., and Gibbons, W. E. Growth curve analyses of follicular growth in the in vitro fertilization program. *Fertil. Steril.* 45:834, 1986.
77. Sathanandan, M., et al. Adjuvant leuprolide in normal, abnormal, and poor responders to controlled ovarian hyperstimulation for in vitro fertilization/gamete intrafallopian transfer. *Fertil. Steril.* 51:998, 1989.
78. Schenker, J. G., and Polishuk, W. Z. The role of prostaglandins in ovarian hyperstimulation syndrome. *Eur. J. Obstet. Gynecol. Reprod. Biol.* 6:47, 1976.
79. Schenker, J. G., and Weinstein, D. Ovarian hyperstimulation syndrome: A current survey. *Fertil. Steril.* 30:25, 1978.
80. Scott, R. T., et al. Follicle-stimulating hormone levels on cycle day 3 are predictive of in vitro fertilization outcome. *Fertil. Steril.* 51:651, 1989.
81. Serafini, P., et al. Occurrence of a spontaneous luteinizing hormone surge in superovulated cycles—predictive value of serum progesterone. *Fertil. Steril.* 49:86, 1988.
82. Sharma, V., et al. Studies on folliculogenesis and in vitro fertilization outcome after the administration of follicle-stimulating hormone at different times during the menstrual cycle. *Fertil. Steril.* 51:298, 1989.
83. Simonetti, S., Veeck, L. L., and Jones, H. W., Jr. Correlation of follicular fluid volume with oocyte morphology from follicles stimulated by human menopausal gonadotropin. *Fertil. Steril.* 44:177, 1985.
84. Speirs, A. L., et al. Analysis of the benefits and risks of multiple embryo transfer. *Fertil. Steril.* 39:468, 1983.
85. Steptoe, P. C., and Edwards, R. G. Birth after the reimplantation of a human embryo. *Lancet* 2:366, 1978.
86. Sterzik, K., et al. In vitro fertilization: The degree of endometrial stimulation. *Fertil. Steril.* 50:457, 1988.
87. Templeton, A., Messinis, I. E., and Baird, D. T. Characteristics of ovarian follicles in spontaneous and stimulated cycles in which there was an endogenous luteinizing hormone surge. *Fertil. Steril.* 46:1113, 1986.
88. Testart, J., et al. Interpretation of plasma luteinizing hormone assay for the collection of mature oocytes from women: Definition of luteinizing hormone surge-initiating rise. *Fertil. Steril.* 36:50, 1981.
89. Thatcher, S. S., et al. A comparison of dosages of norethisterone for synchronization of cycles in a fixed regimen of follicular augmentation and in vitro fertilization. *Fertil. Steril.* 49:848, 1988.

90. Trounson, A. O., et al. Pregnancies in humans by fertilization in vitro and embryo transfer. *Science* 212:682, 1981.

91. Vargyas, J. M., et al. Correlation of ultrasonic measurement of ovarian follicle size and serum estradiol levels in ovulatory patients following clomiphene citrate for in vitro fertilization. *Am. J. Obstet. Gynecol.* 144:569, 1982.

92. Vargyas, J. M., et al. The effect of different methods of ovarian stimulation for human in vitro fertilization and embryo replacement. *Fertil. Steril.* 42:745, 1984.

93. Wang, T-A., et al. The influence of exogenous human chorionic gonadotropin cycles with spontaneous luteinizing hormone surges on the outcome of in vitro fertilization. *Fertil. Steril.* 48:613, 1987.

94. Williams, R. F., and Hodgen, G. D. Disparate effects of human chorionic gonadotropin during the late follicular phase in monkeys: Normal ovulation, follicular atresia, ovarian acyclicity, and hypersecretion of follicle stimulating hormone. *Fertil. Steril.* 33:64, 1980.

95. Wramsby, H., et al. The success rate of in vitro fertilization of human oocytes in relation to the concentrations of different hormones in follicular fluid and peripheral plasma. *Fertil. Steril.* 36:448, 1981.

96. Yee, B., and Vargyas, J. M. Multiple follicle development utilizing combinations of clomiphene citrate and human menopausal gonadotropins. *Clin. Obstet. Gynaecol.* 29:141, 1986.

97. Zimmerman, R., et al. Gonadotropin therapy of female infertility. Analysis of results in 416 cases. *Gynecol. Obstet. Invest.* 14:1, 1982.

# Techniques of Oocyte Retrieval

Bruce L. Tjaden and John A. Rock

Many methods have been described for the recovery/pick-up of oocytes for in vitro fertilization (IVF). Laparoscopic retrieval initially was the procedure of choice and still retains an important role in oocyte recovery; however, this approach has largely been replaced by ultrasound-guided transcutaneous or transvaginal retrieval. Concurrent treatment of pelvic disease (e.g., endometriosis, adhesions, ovarian cysts) done in conjunction with oocyte pick-up and GIFT are reasons that laparoscopy remains and will continue to be an important modality for oocyte pick-up.

Edwards and Steptoe (11) were the first to describe and utilize the laparoscope for egg retrieval. They initially used an aspiration needle with an inside diameter of 1.2 mm. Oocyte recovery was approximately 32%. Lopata and colleagues (9) in 1974 described using an aspiration needle with an inside diameter of 1.4 mm. This improved the recovery rate to approximately 45%. Various different parameters of aspiration needles have been examined as to their effects on recovery rates including material, internal diameter, efficacy of materials lining the needle (e.g., Teflon). There is no consensus in the literature as to the best needle for aspiration; nonetheless, most programs are reporting recovery rates approaching 90–100%. Obvious advantages to laparoscopic retrieval include direct visualization of pelvic contents, direct observation of oocyte recovery, and the opportunity to combine retrieval with operative therapies. A recent report demonstrated the efficacy of combined oocyte retrieval and operative endoscopic treatment of pelvic pathology. Twelve of thirty-nine patients who underwent operative endoscopy at the time of oocyte retrieval for IVF became pregnant during nontreatment cycles within 10 months following operative endoscopy (1). Obvious disadvantages to laparoscopic retrieval include the need for general anesthesia, risks, necessity of operative facilities and ancillary personnel including anesthesia staff. The patient must accept the risks known to be associated with laparoscopy and anesthesia as well as probable greater discomfort/pain to the patient as compared to ultrasound retrieval. In cases of severe pelvic adhesions, the ovaries may not be accessible or visible via the laparoscope as they may be buried beneath adhesions of bowel or omentum, or both.

The first report in the literature of ultrasound-guided retrieval was in *Lancet* in 1981 (7). In this report oocytes were recovered by percutaneous puncture traversing the anterior abdominal wall and the urinary bladder guided by the ultrasound. As a part of the study, patients underwent laparoscopy or laparotomy after the percutaneous puncture and retrieval. Although no pregnancies were reported, no untoward outcomes were identified, and the authors' impression of sonographic-guided puncture was favorable and that it represented an improvement on laparoscopic retrieval especially in women with extensive adhesions. Other favorable reports soon followed. Initially all the reports dealt with percutaneous transabdominal transvesical puncture (Fig. 9-1)(13). Other methods were described including a transurethral approach. In 1983 Gleicher and colleagues reported a transvaginal approach for oocyte recovery (5) (Fig. 9-2)(2). Other reports soon followed confirming the efficacy, safety, and patient acceptance. Initial reports seemed to indicate that the sonographic-guided recovery was less successful than the standard laparoscopic retrieval; however, refined techniques as well as improvements in ultrasound equipment have demonstrated

The opinions expressed herein are those of the authors and are not necessarily those of the United States Air Force or the Department of Defense.

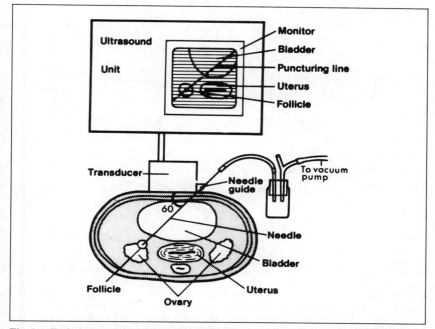

**Fig. 9-1. Technique of transabdominal follicular puncture with ultrasound guidance. (From M. Wikland et al. Collection of human oocytes by the use of sonography.** *Fertil. Steril.* **39:603, 1983. With permission.)**

that recovery rates and pregnancy rates from ultrasonically guided retrievals are equivalent to laparoscopic retrievals.

Complications from transvaginal recovery are infrequent but nonetheless do exist. Howe and colleagues (6) reported on three apparent infectious complications from transvaginal recovery. One patient required total abdominal hysterectomy and bilateral salpingo-ophorectomy as definitive therapy for a tubo-ovarian abscess after failing antibiotics. They use prophylactic antibiotics prior to transvaginal ovum recovery as well as Betadine gel to cleanse the vagina prior to vaginal mucousal puncture. Other authors feel antibiotic coverage is not necessary (8).

Other investigators noted an oocyte culture infection rate of approximately 6%, which is not higher than laparoscopically obtained oocytes and may represent sperm contamination rather than a bacterial inoculum from the vaginal mucosa (4).

## TECHNIQUE FOR LAPAROSCOPIC RECOVERY

An infraumbilical approach is used with one or two additional punctures in the lower abdomen. Laparoscopic retrieval systems today often utilize a two-puncture or a three-puncture system for the insertion of additional instruments. The two-puncture technique uses an offset 10-mm laparoscope with the aspirating needle usually passed through the operating channel. The second puncture (usually a 5-mm sleeve/trocar) is used for placing accessory instruments, e.g., grasping forceps for stabilization of the ovary usually by holding the utero-ovarian ligament or a blunt probe for manipulation of pelvic organs. The three-puncture method is similar to the two-puncture technique; however, an additional 5-mm

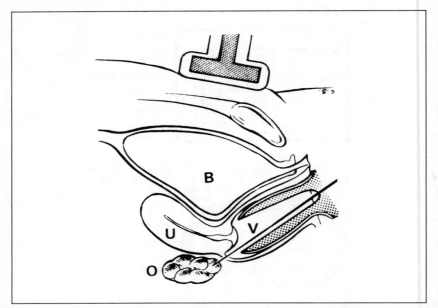

**Fig. 9-2. Technique of transabdominal ultrasound-directed vaginal retrieval. B, bladder; U, uterus; V, vagina; O, ovary. (From P. Dellenbach et al. Transvaginal sonographically controlled puncture for oocyte retrieval. *Fertil. Steril.* 44:656, 1985. With permission.)**

sleeve/trocar can be used to insert instruments for ovarian stabilization or operative procedures, e.g., lysis of adhesions and fulguration of endometriosis. The laparoscopic aspirating needle is 43 cm in length and has a 45-degree bevel at the tip and an internal diameter of 2.16 mm. Of note is the raised band 5 mm from the tip of the needle (Fig. 9-3). The raised band allows the surgeon to determine the depth of penetration into the follicle. The collar furthermore can prevent leakage of fluid from the follicle as it acts to "seal" the puncture site. Under direct visualization follicles are punctured in a systematic manner. After the follicle is punctured, the follicular fluid is aspirated into a delee trap that is handed off to be taken to the lab for evaluation for oocytes. A syringe with Dulbecco's solution is then connected to the needle and the follicle is then flushed. The wash is aspirated into the syringe and likewise taken to the lab for evaluation. A second and occasionally a third wash is performed depending on whether or not the surgeon feels the oocyte has been captured. If the laboratory has identified the egg, no further flushing is carried out. Flushing the follicle more than 2 times has proved to be of little value in our hands. All follicles of 15 mm or greater are aspirated and punctured. Aspiration should be accomplished in a logical systematic fashion as fluid occasionally reaccumulates in the previously punctured follicles, making it difficult to determine which follicle has already been punctured. The contralateral ovary is likewise approached and follicles aspirated. Every attempt to work as efficiently as possible is made to minimize trauma to the uterus and ovaries as well as limiting the amount of anesthetic and carbon dioxide to which the oocytes are exposed.

## TECHNIQUE FOR SONOGRAPHIC OOCYTE RECOVERY

The patient is prepared for oocyte retrieval in a similar fashion as for laparoscopic retrieval. The patient is taken to the operative suite and ultimately placed

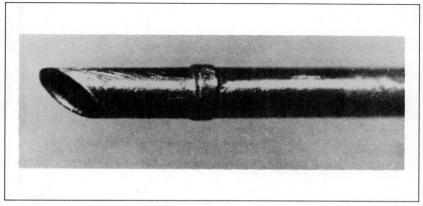

Fig. 9-3. Laparoscopic oocyte aspiration needle (2.16-mm internal diameter) with raised bevel.

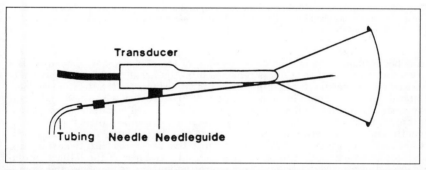

Fig. 9-4. Transvaginal oocyte retrieval technique. (From M. Wikland, L. Enk, and L. Hamberger. Transvesical and transvaginal approaches for the aspiration of follicles by use of ultrasound. In M. Seppala and R. G. Edwards (eds.), *In Vitro Fertilization and Embryo Transfer.* New York: New York Academy of Sciences, 442:182, 1985. With permission.)

in the dorsal lithotomy position. Perineal prep is then carried out. At the Johns Hopkins Hospital, vaginal preparation is done only with normal saline to minimize toxic substances that may interfere with oocyte survival. A sterile condom is placed over the vaginal transducer. A sterile sleeve is placed over the transducer cord and then a second sterile condom is placed over the transducer. To achieve the best sonographic images, care must be taken to ensure that an adequate amount of sonographic gel is placed between the transducer head and the condoms. A sterile speculum is placed in the vagina and a paracervical block is then carried out using 1% Xylocaine. The patient is sometimes lightly sedated with Fentanyl and occasionally Surital by the anesthesia staff. Most patients do surprisingly well with infiltration of local anesthetics, and most require little if any intravenous sedation. The covered sonographic transducer is fit with the appropriate needle guide and placed in the vagina (Fig. 9-4)(12). Transvaginal scanning is then performed for orientation, localization, and counting of potential follicles, as well as the relative location of other important pelvic structures, e.g., uterus, major blood vessels, psoas muscle. The needle is then placed through the needle guide. On puncturing the vaginal mucosa, the tip of the needle, which

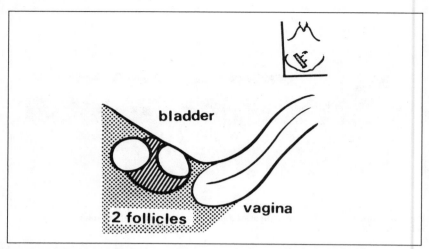

**Fig. 9-5. Identification of follicles with transvaginal scan. (From P. Dellenbach et al. Transvaginal sonographically controlled follicle puncture for oocyte retrieval. *Fertil. Steril.* 44:656, 1985. With permission.)**

has been made more echogenic by etching of the surface, can be seen on the ultrasound screen. The stylet is removed from the needle and a 5-ml syringe is placed on the needle. By manipulating the transducer with anterior-posterior, lateral, and rotational movements (Fig. 9-5)(2), the ovary with the follicles can be easily identified. Follicular puncture is then carried out under direct sonographic guidance. A steady puncture is preferred. Once the follicle is punctured, gentle aspiration is applied with the syringe and the follicular fluid is aspirated. Care should be taken to avoid excessive negative pressures with the aspirating syringe to avoid trauma to the oocytes. Usually collapse of the follicle can be seen on the ultrasound screen. The aspirating syringe is removed and immediately replaced with a syringe containing Dulbecco's solution. The follicle is then "washed" and the irrigating solution aspirated. The follicle is usually flushed a second time and perhaps a third. The follicular fluid-aspirate and each wash is separately marked and immediately taken to the lab for evaluation for oocytes. The needle is then removed from the follicle (but not removed from the ovary), then repositioned in an attempt to isolate and align the next follicle. All successive punctures are accomplished in the same manner as the first. Aspiration of follicles should be carried out in a logical, orderly fashion from one side of the ovary to the other. Follicles punctured may reaccumulate fluid and may after a short while appear to be unpunctured follicles. Therefore an orderly progression is best to maximize oocyte recovery and minimize potential confusion. The follicular fluid is usually a clear straw color; occasionally it is slightly blood tinged. Follicle washes are slightly more blood tinged. A dark red aspirated fluid indicates that a follicle has been previously punctured and reaccumulated. After all follicles have been aspirated from one ovary, the needle is removed from the ovary and subsequently from the vaginal mucosa. A "needle wash" is then carried out by flushing the needle with Dulbecco's solution. The fluid is sent to the lab for evaluation of oocytes. Occasionally an oocyte is recovered from this procedure. The contralateral ovary is then identified and positioned with respect to the ultrasound screen. The needle is replaced within the needle guide, the vaginal mucosa is punctured, and the stylet is removed. Follicular puncture is then carried out. On completion of the procedure, the needle and the transducer are removed. A speculum exam is then carried out to ensure that

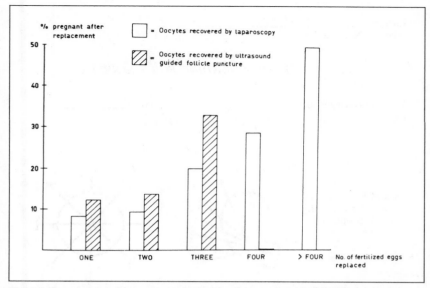

**Fig. 9-6. Comparison of pregnancy rates with ultrasound-guided or laparoscopic retrieval (From W. Feichtinger and P. Kempter. Laparoscopic or ultrasonically guided follicle aspiration for in vitro fertilization?** *J. In Vitro Fert. Embryo Trans.***, 1:244, 1984. With permission.)**

there is no bleeding from the mucosal puncture sites. Any bleeding is usually minimal and can usually be controlled with gentle tamponading pressure with a gauze pad.

The patient is placed in the dorsal supine position and subsequently transferred to the recovery room where she is observed for 2 hours. Usually, however, recovery time is less than 1 hour. Most patients require only slight sedation for the procedure and are usually awake and alert enough to view the process on the ultrasound screen and thus require only minimal amount of time for recovery. Patients are discharged home only after vitals have been observed to be stable and the patient is fully alert and oriented. All are given explicit instructions to notify the staff of any complications or apparent problems.

Eighty-five to ninety-five percent of follicles yield an oocyte when laparoscopic recovery is utilized; a 75–85% recovery rate has been achieved with sonographic recovery. Fertilization and pregnancy rates are similar for both groups, approaching 15–18% per embryo transfer. One unrandomized comparison of the two methods found a higher pregnancy rate in the ultrasound-guided group, when up to three embryos were replaced (Fig. 9-6) (3).

The literature overwhelmingly supports vaginal ovum recovery as the procedure of choice for most IVF patients. Morbidity is low, patient acceptance is high, cost is less, and success rates are equal to laparoscopic retrieval. A recent report could find no deleterious effects of ultrasound on human oocytes, thus supporting ultrasound over laparoscopy for most IVF patients (10).

## TECHNIQUES OF EMBRYO TRANSFER

The procedure of embryo transfer itself is usually accomplished with a minimal amount of difficulty. In the laboratory the embryo(s) is loaded into an open-

Patient _____

History No. _____

### UTERINE SOUNDING FOR TRANSFER

Uterine cavity size:    inches _____  cm _____

Position:    Ant _____  Mid _____  Retro _____

Axis of Uterine Cavity
(Note by checking
off appropriate
arrows)

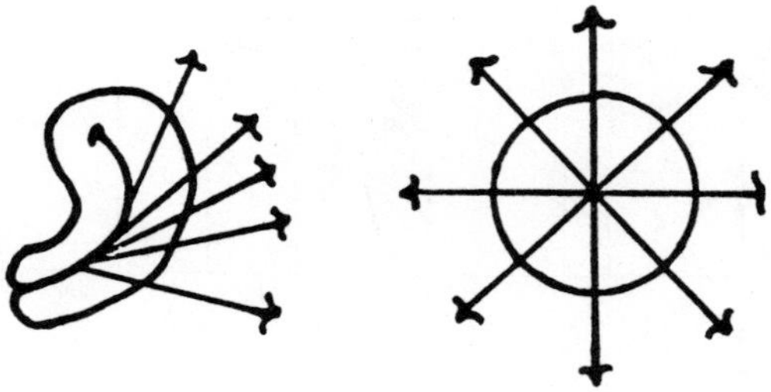

Examiner:    _____

Date:    _____

Fig 9-7. Uterine sounding for embryo transfer.

ended Teflon catheter in the following fashion: 5-$\mu$l media, 5-$\mu$l air, embryos, 5-$\mu$l air, 5-$\mu$l media. The catheter is then taken immediately to the embryo transfer room where the patient is already in the lithotomy position and prepared for the procedure to be performed. Patient preparation for the procedure involves placing the patient on a suitable adjustable examining table and placement of a sterile speculum into the patient's vagina. The cervix and vagina are then cleansed with warm Dulbecco's solution. A cervical tenaculum is available if needed. The embryos are then brought to the examining room during which time the Teflon catheter is placed through the cervix into the uterine fundus and the embryo is gently deposited with a slow depression on the plunger of a 1-cc tuberculin syringe. Approximately 0.5-cc of air is required in the tuberculin syringe for complete depression of the plunger.

The embryo transfer may be accomplished easily with placement of the catheter into the plane of the uterine axis. During the ovulation induction a test pass with the Teflon catheter is performed prior to oocyte retrieval. The axis of the uterus is then noted on the patient's ovulation induction sheet, allowing the surgeon to perform the embryo transfer according to these guidelines (Fig. 9-7). If the patient has a tortuous cervical canal, a metal catheter may be used for embryo transfer.

Although the embryo transfer is the simplest procedure associated with IVF, it is the procedure associated with the success rate of each individual cycle. An increasing number of embryos are associated with a higher pregnancy rate

Table 9-1. Pregnancy rates versus number of embryos transferred

| Number of embryos transferred | Pregnancy rate (%) |
| --- | --- |
| 1 | 9–10 |
| 2 | 12–15 |
| 3 | 15–20 |
| 4 or more | 20–25 |

(Table 9-1). This explains the rationale for increasing the number of fertilizable oocytes to be recruited and fertilized.

Other aspects of IVF, namely ovulation induction, are associated with a 93–95% success rate in recruiting multiple oocytes. The oocyte retrieval is also associated with a 89–95% success rate in obtaining oocytes. Fertilization rates are approximately 79–85% with mature oocytes; however, after embryo transfer, pregnancy rates are in the range of 15–20%. This percentage may be associated with a number of factors.

Suggested problems associated with the embryo transfer stage of IVF include asynchrony of the uterine endometrium possibly induced by exogenous gonadotropins. It has been postulated that the endometrium may be altered by gonadotropin therapy and thus not be as receptive to implantation as would the natural cycle. Progesterone support for this luteal "defect" has been discussed in Chap. 8 with respect to the luteal phase of the in vitro cycle. Asynchrony may also exist between in vitro embryo development and embryo development in vivo. Human embryos reach the blastocyst stage in vivo at approximately 100 hours compared to 120 hours with in vitro incubation. Possibly this lag in embryo development is associated with the percentage of successful implantations associated with any single in vitro cycle. Also the receptivity of any one human cycle to the establishment of pregnancy may only be 20–25% per cycle since natural pregnancy rates appear to approach a similar statistical change of implantation according to life table analysis.

## REFERENCES

1. Damewood M. D., and Rock J. A. Treatment independent pregnancy with operative laparoscopy for endometriosis in an in vitro fertilization program. *Fertil. Steril.* 50:463, 1988.
2. Dellenbach, P., et al. Transvaginal sonographically controlled follicle puncture for oocyte retrieval. *Fertil. Steril.* 44:656, 1985.
3. Feichtinger, W., and Kemeter, P. Laparoscopic or ultrasonically guided follicle aspiration for in vitro fertilization? *J. In Vitro Fert. Embryo Transf.* 1:244, 1984.
4. Feichtinger, W., and Kemeter, P. Transvaginal sector scan sonography for needle guided transvaginal follicle aspiration and other applications in gynecologic routine and research. *Fertil. Steril.* 45:5, 1986.
5. Gleicher, N., et al. Egg retrieval for IVF by sonographically controlled vaginal culdocentesis. *Lancet* 27 Aug. 2:508–509, 1983.
6. Howe, R. S., et al. Pelvic infection after transvaginal ultrasound-guided ovum retrieval. *Fertil. Steril.* 49:4, 1988.
7. Lenz, S., Lavritsen, J. G., and Kjellow, M. Collection of human oocyte for IVF by ultrasonically guided follicular puncture. *Lancet* 1:1163, 1981.
8. Lenz, S., Leeton J., and Renou, P. Transvaginal recovery of oocytes for IVF using vaginal ultrasound. *J. In Vitro Fert. Embryo Transf.* 4:1, 1987.
9. Lopata, A., et al. Collection of human oocytes with laparoscopy and laparotomy. *Fertil. Steril.* 25:1030, 1974.
10. Mahadevan, M., et al. Evidence for an absence of deleterious effects of ultrasound on human oocytes. *J. In Vitro Fert. Embryo Transf.* 4:5, 1987.

11. Steptoe, P. C., and Edwards, R. G. Laparoscopic recovery of preovulatory human oocytes after priming of ovaries with gonadotropins. *Lancet* 1:683, 1970.
12. Wikland, M., Enk, L., and Hamberger, L. Transvesical and Transvaginal Approaches for the Aspiration of Follicles by Use of Ultrasound. In M. Seppala and R. G. Edwards (eds.), *In Vitro Fertilization and Embryo Transfer*. New York: New York Academy of Sciences, 442:182, 1985.
13. Wikland, M., et al. Collection of human oocytes by the use of sonography. *Fertil. Steril.* 39:603, 1983.

# Laboratory

# Laboratory Preparation for Human IVF-ET

Meriella J. Hubbard and Leslie Weikert

## ORGANIZATION AND QUALITY CONTROL IN THE IN VITRO FERTILIZATION LABORATORY AREAS

In order to maximize the success of any in vitro fertilization (IVF) program, careful attention to sterility and routine quality control procedures is critical in all laboratory areas and with all laboratory procedures (4,6). Currently, our program has two laboratory areas for human IVF and embryo transfer (IVF-ET): an oocyte/embryo culture laboratory and a media and semen preparation laboratory. In the latter, the glassware required for IVF-ET is washed, cleaned, and sterilized only by IVF personnel using an acceptable and standardized protocol. Our standardized protocol includes washing the glassware in tissue culture detergent, rinsing the glassware extremely well with double-glass distilled water, packaging, and autoclaving the glassware and any other "autoclavable" equipment required or used in the IVF procedure. The ultrasound needles used are large-gauge echo-tip disposable needles (Cook Obgyn No. KDSN-172501), and the laparoscope needles used are disposable Norfolk aspiration needles for laparoscopy (Cook Obgyn No. KNOAN-124300). This standardized protocol minimizes the possibility of contamination of the equipment with toxic substances or residues that may be left during routine hospital washing and sterilization.

In the oocyte/embryo culture laboratory, scrub clothing, complete with mask, hat, and shoe covers is required. Prior to any IVF-ET activity in either lab, all personnel thoroughly scrub their hands with Exidine-4 scrub solution.

Furthermore, in both lab areas the following general quality control rules are followed: (1) all equipment and work surfaces are wiped down with 70% ethyl alcohol daily; (2) air-conditioned air is prefiltered and supplied under positive pressure; (3) laminar flow hoods, which are certified annually, are turned on to provide additional room-air filtration; however, the hoods are turned off in the oocyte/embryo culture laboratory during oocyte and embryo manipulation because of the rapid pH changes in the insemination media and growth media and temperature fluctuation of the warming plates caused by the rapidly circulating air in the laminar flow hood system; (4) media preparation, dilutions, pipetting, and transfers are done under horizontal laminar flow hoods; (5) ultraviolet lights, located near or in each laminar flow hood, which reduce the presence of microbiologic contaminants, are inspected regularly and turned on ONLY after IVF personnel have left the lab areas; (6) incubators are regularly "disassembled," and all trays, side panels, shelves, and water pans are washed and sterilized. Furthermore, the outside glass and door panels of the incubators are wiped with 70% ethyl alcohol. The water jackets lining the incubators are flushed out annually and replaced with sterile distilled water. Finally, carbon dioxide concentrations are tested regularly with a fyrite indicator, and the carbon dioxide alarm system, which is attached to the incubators, is checked regularly; and (7) gloves are never worn to manipulate oocytes/embryos due to toxicity and a limitation of dexterity; however, gloves are worn and rinsed for the preparation of the semen sample.

## PREPARATION OF CULTURE MEDIUM AND SERUM SUPPLEMENT

Quality control standards are also followed for the preparation of culture media and serum supplements used for semen preparation, follicular aspiration, oocyte culture, embryo culture, and embryo transfer.

## Protein Supplements

Our program currently uses pooled male serum as the serum supplement in the preparation of the insemination medium and growth medium.

The serum is obtained from young, healthy men. The blood is drawn into a 60-ml syringe (Becton-Dickinson) using a 19-gauge butterfly needle (Abbott Hospitals). Approximately 100-ml of blood is drawn from each male volunteer. The blood is poured into 50-ml Falcon No. 2070 centrifuge tubes and allowed to clot, and the serum is separated by centrifugation. Usually, multiple centrifugations are necessary to remove formed particles or gels. The serum is then heat inactivated for 45 minutes at 56°C, filter sterilized (0.2 $\mu$m), and frozen as separate lots at $-20$°C. Prior to heat inactivation, an aliquot of each male serum is separated out and tested for human immunodeficiency virus and hepatitis. Furthermore, each serum is tested for embryo toxicity using the mouse embryo system in which each serum is evaluated for its ability to enhance or promote the development of mouse embryos from the two-cell stage to the blastocyst stage. The blastocyst stage is observed after approximately 75 hours of culture; however, serum that inhibits embryo development can, in most cases, be identified after only 24 hours of culture (7). Only those serums that pass the above tests are pooled, and the new pooled serum is retested again for embryo toxicity.

## Culture Medium

Presently our laboratory uses two culture medias: Ham's F-10 (Gibco No. 430-1200) and Dulbecco's phosphate buffered saline (Gibco No. 3104287). The Ham's F-10 is used for sperm washing, oocyte culture, embryo culture, and embryo transfer; the Dulbecco's phosphate buffered saline is used at the time of oocyte retrieval to flush the aspiration needles prior to and after follicular aspiration and for flushing the follicles after they have been aspirated. The Ham's F-10 is supplied in a powdered form and is reconstituted in our laboratory. The Dulbecco's, however, is already prepared and commercially available. Both culture media are purchased in great quantities, and each group of culture media comes from the same quality control lot number assigned to it by Gibco. Prior to their use in human IVF-ET, each media is tested for embryo toxicity in the mouse embryo system as described earlier. At the time of quality control testing, each media is adjusted to an osmolarity of 280 mOsm/kg with bottled sterile distilled water purchased from the hospital pharmacy and pertaining to a single lot number. Furthermore, 0.7 ml of reconstituted penicillin/streptomycin (Gibco No. 600-5145) is added to each 100 ml of media. Insemination medium and growth medium are prepared by adding 10% pooled male serum to each one. Approximately 1.0-ml of either insemination media or growth media is placed in the inner well of a Falcon No. 3037 organ culture dish; 3-ml of "plain" media is placed in the outer well. The media is allowed to equilibrate for a minimum of 6 hours in a 5% carbon dioxide and air environment prior to its use in either the mouse embryo test or in the human IVF-ET culture system.

After all of the quality control tests have been performed, and both culture media and serum supplements pass, the laboratory personnel, using sterile technique, make up heparinized phosphate buffered saline and the insemination media with 10% male serum approximately 17 hours prior to oocyte retrieval. The growth media, with 10% male serum, is made up at approximately the time the oocytes are inseminated. Both media are pipetted into organ culture dishes that are appropriately labeled with the patient's name. Prior to oocyte retrieval, laboratory personnel keep close contact with the progress of the patient's induced multiple follicular development through ultrasound and estradiol levels. This information allows the laboratory personnel to plan for the appropriate number of organ culture dishes with insemination media that may be required at the time of oocyte pick-up.

## SEMEN PREPARATION FOR IVF

### Background

As a routine method for evaluating the husband of a woman undergoing IVF and *prior* to the induction of ovarian hyperstimulation for IVF, a basic semen analysis is performed. The semen sample is collected by masturbation after at least 3 days of abstinence from ejaculation. The semen analysis includes microbiologic culture for *Mycoplasma, Ureaplasma urealyticum,* and *Chlamydia trachomatis;* evaluation of liquefaction; viscosity; volume; sperm and leukocyte concentration; and motility and sperm morphology. Also, when indicated, a check for antisperm antibodies is performed. The techniques used to assess sperm quality are based on those of the World Health Organization's *Laboratory Manual for the Examination of Human Semen and Semen-Cervical Mucus Interaction* (1).

Following the evaluation of the semen sample, if a problem or a combination of problems exists such as low count, abnormal motility, a high percentage of abnormal sperm or a high concentration of acellular debris, or a combination of these, additional manipulations such as using a discontinuous Percoll gradient (2) may be necessary in order to enhance the recovery of a population of highly motile and progressive spermatozoa.

### Processing the Semen Sample for IVF

Approximately 2½ hours prior to insemination, the husband is instructed to produce a semen sample by masturbation. He has been asked to abstain from ejaculation for 3–5 days, void urine, wash his hands before masturbating, and avoid using any form of unnatural lubrication. The semen specimen is collected in a sterile plastic container (specimen containers No. C8827-4 from American Scientific Products). He is asked to label the container with his name and his wife's name. The semen sample is allowed to liquefy for approximately 30 minutes in a 37°C warming oven. Once liquefaction appears to be complete, the specimen cup is gently rotated to mix the semen. The entire ejaculate is transferred to a labeled sterile 15-ml centrifuge tube (Falcon No. 2095) using a sterile 1-, 5-, or 10-ml pipette (Falcon No. 7521, No. 7543, and No. 7551, respectively). The sample is mixed well by gently pipetting it up and down. At this time the sample is checked for volume, color, and liquefaction. If the sample has many gelatinous clumps, the specimen is allowed to sit for approximately 5 minutes. During this time, the clumps settle to the bottom of the tube and the semen-supernatant is transferred to another labeled 15-ml centrifuge tube (5). The sample is again mixed well with a pipette. Using a 20-μl pipetman, 10-μl of the *well*-mixed semen is placed on a clean glass microscope slide, covered with a 22-mm coverslip, and examined under a magnification of 400× using a phase contrast Nikon microscope (40× objective and 10× eyepiece). One hundred spermatozoa are counted twice to assess motility and forward progression. Furthermore, a visual assessment of sperm concentration is performed in order to determine the dilution of the semen sample necessary to formally assess sperm concentration. Depending on the specimen, an aliquot of well-mixed semen is mixed with an aliquot of sperm fixative (10 ml of 35% formalin in 1000 ml of distilled water) in a small 12 × 75-mm test tube and gently vortexed. Using a Pasteur pipette, a small drop of the well-mixed diluted semen is applied to the outer edges of the coverslip on each side of the central trough of a Neubauer Counting Chamber (hemocytometer). The preparation is left for approximately 5 minutes to allow the cells to settle. Then each chamber is viewed microscopically at a magnification of 400×, and the number of spermatozoa in five large squares of the chamber is counted. Sperm concentration is calculated in the following way:

Average number of sperm counted × dilution factor × 5 (0.20 mm is area in which sperm are counted) × 10 (depth of μm of counting chamber) × 1000 (to convert mm to ml) = number of sperm per ml.

After motility and sperm concentration have been determined, the sample is diluted and gently mixed with at least 3 times its original volume of insemination media. The insemination media consists of Ham's F-10 supplemented with 10% pooled male heat-inactivated serum. If the initial volume of the liquefied specimen plus insemination media exceeds the capacity of the 15-ml centrifuge tube, then the specimen is split into the appropriate number of tubes needed to ensure proper washing. The diluted semen sample is generally divided among two sterile 15-ml centrifuge tubes and centrifuged at 146 × gravity for 10 minutes. Then, the supernatants are discarded using a sterile transfer pipette (Samco No. 202-1S). Each pellet is resuspended in 3 ml of fresh insemination media and centrifuged again for 10 minutes at 146 × g. Once again the supernatants are discarded. Each pellet is gently layered with 0.5 ml of insemination media and incubated at 37° C in a humidified atmosphere of 5% carbon dioxide in air for 1 hour.

After 1 hour, the top 0.4 ml of insemination media containing the highly motile spermatozoa from each tube is combined and transferred to another sterile labeled 15-ml centrifuge tube. The supernatant is analyzed to determine sperm concentration, motility, and forward progression. An aliquot of 100 μl of culture media containing approximately 100,000 motile spermatozoa is added to each culture dish housing a "mature" oocyte. Therefore, in general, a concentration of 1 × 10 motile spermatozoa per ml is prepared for the insemination of 10 oocytes. After the sperm suspension has been added, any remaining portion of the sperm suspension is incubated overnight and used to check sperm viability as a measure of quality control (Fig. 10-1).

## OOCYTE RETRIEVAL

Oocyte pick-up is performed either by laparoscopy or ultrasound-guided transvaginal aspiration. In either method, suction may be applied to the aspiration system by a foot-operated Craft suction machine set at 60 mm of mercury. The follicle contents are aspirated into a warmed Argyle-DeLee suction trap tube or a 5-ml syringe that is sequentially numbered in order to keep track of the number of follicles punctured per ovary. Following aspiration, follicles are irrigated and flushed with 3-ml of heparinized Dulbecco's phosphate buffered saline. As soon as aspiration is complete, the DeLee trap is quickly transferred to the adjacent culture laboratory. There, the collected follicular fluid is immediately checked for pH, color, and volume and then poured into a Falcon No. 3002 petri dish. The follicular volumes obtained may range from 2–8 ml. The follicular fluid is examined for the presence of an oocyte. Mature oocytes with expanded cumulus can be located very quickly. A quick microscopic evaluation of the maturity and morphology of the oocyte is done at this time. The presence of either sheets of granulosa cells; a dispersed and uniform cumulus; adequate stretchability of its matrix or a viscous follicular fluid, or both, *suggests* the oocyte is "mature" (3); however, the observation of any of the listed criteria does not necessarily imply the identification of a "mature healthy oocyte."

Whether an oocyte is or is not found in the follicular aspirate, the corresponding follicle wash, obtained by flushing the follicle with 3-ml of heparinized Dulbecco's phosphate buffer saline, is examined for the possible presence of an oocyte. Also, after aspiration is complete, all of the needles used during the procedure are thoroughly flushed and the "needle wash" is examined for the presence of oocytes.

Using a sterile Pasteur capillary pipette attached to a small latex bulb, the oocyte is first "washed" in plain Ham's F-10 media in the outer well of a Falcon No. 3037 culture dish. After the wash, the oocyte is transferred to the inner well, which contains fresh Ham's F-10 media with 10% heat-treated male serum,

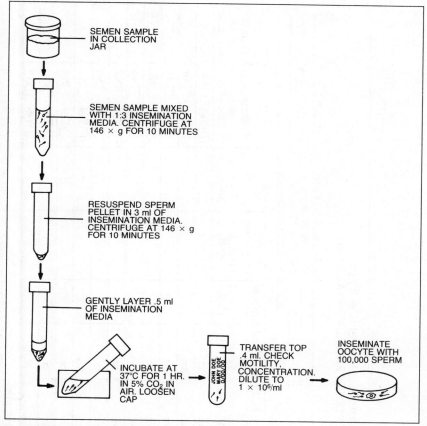

**Fig. 10-1. Steps in the semen preparation for human IVF.**

and placed in a 37°C incubator with an atmosphere of 5% carbon dioxide and air (8). The oocytes that are classified as "mature" at the time of pick-up are incubated for 3–8 hours. After the predetermined incubation period is up, an aliquot of 100 μl of culture media containing approximately 100,000 motile spermatozoa is added to each culture dish containing a mature oocyte. The oocyte and sperm suspension is placed back into the 5% carbon dioxide incubator.

An initial record of each puncture, follicular fluid volume and color, oocyte found, and laboratory handling of the specimens is maintained (Fig. 10-2).

### Evaluation of Fertilization and Embryo Development

Approximately 15–18 hours after insemination, the oocytes are examined for morphologic "indications" of fertilization. Some of these indications include (1) the formation and extrusion of the second polar body; (2) the presence of two pronuclei; (3) the cytoplasm of the egg contracted away from the zona pellucida; and (4) normal cleavage. In the event that cells covering the conceptus obscure examination, they are mechanically removed by gently pipetting them to remove any remaining cumulus or by using a 1-ml syringe that is attached to a 25-gauge needle (Becton-Dickinson). Furthermore, if at the time of examination

**JOHNS HOPKINS HOSPITAL**
**OOCYTE RETRIEVAL—DATA SHEET**

Patient _____
Date Retrieved _____
Technician _____
Retriever (Phys.) _____

Coelomic Fluid pH _____
Culture Medium _____
Diluting Medium _____
Foll. Flush Medium _____

Day hCG _____
Time hCG _____
Anesthetic _____
$CO_2$ Time _____

| Ovary (R.L.) | Follicle | Oocyte # | Grade (Poor, Fair, Good) | Follicular Fluid Aspirate | | | | | | Time to Incubator | Sample Saved (FF-Cells) | Sample Storage Location |
| --- | --- | --- | --- | --- | --- | --- | --- | --- | --- | --- | --- | --- |
| | | | | Time to Lab | Initial Volume | Volume of Dil. | Color | Granulosa Cells | | | | |
| | | | | | cc | cc | | | | | ☐Yes ☐No | |
| | | | | | cc | cc | | | | | ☐Yes ☐No | |
| | | | | | cc | cc | | | | | ☐Yes ☐No | |
| | | | | | cc | cc | | | | | ☐Yes ☐No | |
| | | | | | cc | cc | | | | | ☐Yes ☐No | |
| | | | | | cc | cc | | | | | ☐Yes ☐No | |
| | | | | | cc | cc | | | | | ☐Yes ☐No | |
| | | | | | cc | cc | | | | | ☐Yes ☐No | |
| | | | | | cc | cc | | | | | ☐Yes ☐No | |
| | | | | | cc | cc | | | | | ☐Yes ☐No | |
| | | | | | cc | cc | | | | | ☐Yes ☐No | |

Fig. 10-2. Data sheet used to record the steps of oocyte retrieval.

**JOHNS HOPKINS HOSPITAL**
OOCYTE/EMBRYO DESCRIPTION SHEET

Patient _____
Date of Retrieval _____
Patient Group _____

Evaluator _____
Time Retrieval Completed _____
Patient Code _____

| Oocyte | Day | T | Day | T | Day | T | Day | T | Day | T |
|---|---|---|---|---|---|---|---|---|---|---|
| | ☐GV ☐PB ☐PN ☐EMB | | ☐GV ☐PB ☐PN ☐EMB | | ☐GV ☐PB ☐PN ☐EMB | | ☐GV ☐PB ☐PN ☐EMB | | ☐GV ☐PB ☐PN ☐EMB | |
| Remarks → | | | | | | | | | | |

| Oocyte | Day | T | Day | T | Day | T | Day | T | Day | T |
|---|---|---|---|---|---|---|---|---|---|---|
| | ☐GV ☐PB ☐PN ☐EMB | | ☐GV ☐PB ☐PN ☐EMB | | ☐GV ☐PB ☐PN ☐EMB | | ☐GV ☐PB ☐PN ☐EMB | | ☐GV ☐PB ☐PN ☐EMB | |
| Remarks → | | | | | | | | | | |

| Oocyte | Day | T | Day | T | Day | T | Day | T | Day | T |
|---|---|---|---|---|---|---|---|---|---|---|
| | ☐GV ☐PB ☐PN ☐EMB | | ☐GV ☐PB ☐PN ☐EMB | | ☐GV ☐PB ☐PN ☐EMB | | ☐GV ☐PB ☐PN ☐EMB | | ☐GV ☐PB ☐PN ☐EMB | |
| Remarks → | | | | | | | | | | |

Fig. 10-3. Data sheet used to record the progress of the oocytes and embryos.

---

### JOHNS HOPKINS HOSPITAL
### EMBRYO TRANSFER SHEET

Patient _____     Patient Group _____
Date of Transfer _____     Time of Transfer _____
Physician _____     Technician _____

#### Specimen Data

Embryos Transferred _____     Volume _____
Transfer Medium _____     Time Loaded _____

#### Equipment Data

Catheter _____
Instrument Used on Cervix: ☐Yes ☐No

#### Procedural Complications

Pain/Cramps: ☐Yes ☐No
Blood on Catheter: ☐Yes ☐No

Comments
_____
_____
_____
_____
_____
_____
_____
_____
_____
_____
_____
_____

Fig. 10-4. Data sheet used to record the embryo transfer.

we are unable to determine any positive evidence of fertilization, the oocytes are transferred to fresh insemination media and reinseminated.

If fertilization is observed, the zygote or pronucleated oocyte is evaluated (Fig. 10-3) and then transferred to growth media for further development. As a rule, the oocytes are firmly attached to the dish by the corona or cumulus cells. Therefore, gentle pipetting is usually necessary to loosen the oocyte from the dish in order to transfer it to growth media (9). The growth media is prepared at the time the oocytes are inseminated in order to allow the media to equilibrate prior to their transfer. The embryos are then placed back into the 5% carbon dioxide incubator under the same conditions used earlier during insemination.

The fertilized oocyte is then observed 38–40 hours after insemination for cleavage, dividing cells of approximately equal size, a homogenous appearance, or a combination of these. After examination and evaluation, the embryos are placed back into the 5% carbon dioxide incubator. At this time, the ET is scheduled. Generally, ET is scheduled 43–48 hours following insemination (Fig. 10-4).

Prior to the actual ET, the embryos are examined for the last time, and only those embryos that are judged to be developing normally are placed together in fresh growth media in a Falcon No. 3037 culture dish. Shortly thereafter, the embryo transfer apparatus, which includes a tomcat catheter and a 1-ml syringe, is assembled. Using sterile technique, 1-ml of fresh growth media is drawn up into the 1-ml syringe. The syringe is connected to the tomcat and the catheter is flushed. The tomcat is then loaded in the following sequence: 5 μl of media, small plug of air, 20 μl of media containing the embryos, another plug of air, and finally, 5 μl of media. The loaded catheter is then carefully handed to the physician. The catheter is passed through the internal cervical os and into the uterus. The contents of the catheter are expelled into the uterus. The catheter is removed and quickly returned to the laboratory and thoroughly flushed with culture medium to ensure the successful transfer of the embryos.

## REFERENCES

1. Belsey, M. A., et al. *Laboratory Manual for the Examination of Human Semen and Semen-Cervical Mucus Interaction.* Switzerland: World Health Organization, 1980.
2. Berger, T., Marrs, R. P., and Moyer, D. L. Comparison of techniques for selection of motile spermatozoa. *Fertil. Steril.* 43:268, 1985.
3. Edwards, R. G., et al. Observations on preovulatory human ovarian follicles and their aspirates. *Br. J. Obstet. Gynaecol.* 87:769, 1980.
4. Jones, H. W., Jr., et al. The program for in vitro fertilization at Norfolk. *Fertil. Steril.* 38:14, 1985.
5. Mahadevan, M., and Baker, G. Assessment and preparation of semen for in vitro fertilization. In C. Wood and A. Trounson (eds.), *Clinical In Vitro Fertilization.* Berlin: Springer-Verlag, 1983. Pp. 83–97.
6. Quinn, P., et al. Culture factors in relation to the success of human in vitro fertilization and embryo transfer. *Fertil. Steril.* 41:202, 1984.
7. Shirley, B., et al. Effects of human serum and plasma on development of mouse embryos in culture media. *Fertil. Steril.* 43:129, 1985.
8. Veek, L. L. Laboratory procedures and responsibilities associated with an in vitro fertilization program. *Infertility* 6:319, 1983.
9. Wortham, J. W. E., Jr., and Witmyer, J. Laboratory aspects in in vitro fertilization. In S. J. Behrman, R. W. Kistner, and G. W. Patton, Jr. (eds.), *Progress in Infertility.* Boston: Little, Brown, 1988. Pp. 601–619.

# Appendix 10-1. Start-up Laboratory Equipment and Supplies

## EQUIPMENT

| Item | *Approximate Cost (1990) |
|---|---|
| Bellco horizontal laminar flow hood No. 8030-76300 (6 ft) | $4000.00 |
| Nikon Diaphot inverted microscope (include 35-mm camera, phase accessories) | 8500.00 |
| Nikon SMZ-10 stereomicroscope with accessories | 2500.00 |
| Forma $CO_2$, water jacketed incubator No. 3326 (include humidity pans) | 3000.00 |
| Two-gauge $CO_2$ regulator | 120.00 |
| Advanced Instruments freezing point determination osmometer No. 3W | 3200.00 |
| Corning pH meter No. 130 | 1100.00 |
| Microelectrode No. MI-410, Microelectrodes, Inc. | 100.00 |
| IEC centrifuge, model HNS-II (include rotor, trunnions, and shields to accommodate Falcon No. 2095 centrifuge tubes) | 1700.00 |
| Labline slide warming tray | 300.00 |
| Precision dual unit water bath | 1000.00 |
| Bacharach Instruments fyrite $CO_2$ analyzer | 150.00 |
| G.E. 1/3 horse power vacuum filter pump | 450.00 |
| Sartorius analytical balance | 4800.00 |
| Refrigerator/freezer | 1000.00 |
| Forma ultra low temperature freezer | 6600.00 |
| Millipore complete water purification system (include final UF cartridge) with accessories | 9000.00 |

## ADDITIONAL EQUIPMENT FOR MAXIMUM EFFICIENCY

| Item | *Approximate Cost (1990) |
|---|---|
| Second horizontal laminar flow hood | 4000.00 |
| Second forma incubator | 3000.00 |
| Additional backup microscopes | 7500–9000.00 |
| IBM PCAT computerization system | 10,000.00 |
| Backup suggested for all quality control and routine smaller equipment | |

*Costs are *approximations* only

## SUPPLIES

| Item | Item No. | Company |
|---|---|---|
| Specimen containers | C8827-4 | American Scientific Products |
| Falcon tissue culture flasks | T4162-25 | " |
| 5¾" Dispo pipettes | P5205-2 | " |
| 9" Dispo pipettes | P5210-2 | " |
| Falcon culture tubes (2003) | T1343-1 | " |
| Falcon culture tubes (2001) | T1342-1 | " |
| 15-ml Falcon centrifuge tubes (2095) | C3978-15 | " |
| 50-ml Falcon centrifuge tubes (2070) | C3978-50 | " |
| Falcon 10-ml sterile pipettes (7551) | P4675-110 | " |
| Falcon 1-ml sterile pipettes (7521) | P4675-11X | " |

| | | |
|---|---|---|
| Falcon culture dishes (3002) | T4155-2 | " |
| Falcon organ culture dishes (3037) | | " |
| Nalgene filter units (500 ml) | F3200-5 | " |
| Nalgene filter units (115 ml) | F3200-1 | " |
| Rubber bulbs | R5002-2 | " |
| Clinitrol 290 osmometer standard | N6025-8 | " |
| Microscope slides | M6157 | " |
| Microscope slide coverslips | M6022-10 | " |
| Dichrol solution | C6355 | " |
| Dispo pipette wrap | P5330 | " |
| Revco freezer boxes | R4091-15 | " |
| Revco box dividers | R4091-17 | " |
| pH buffer, 7.0 | H7590-7 | " |
| pH buffer, 8.0 | H7590-8 | " |
| MLA pipette tips | P5064-902 | " |
| MLA pipette tips | P5064-903P | " |
| MLA automatic pipetters (various sizes) | P5064(+size)D | " |
| Falcon pipet-aid, automatic pipetter | P4570-2 | " |
| Hemacytometer | B3180-1 | " |
| ¾″ white tape | L1607-2 | " |
| 50 cc B/D syringes | | Hospital supply |
| 16-gauge Yale needles, 1½″ | | " |
| 19-gauge Yale needles, 1½″ | | " |
| Autoclave indicator tape | | " |
| Tuberculin syringes | | " |
| Technical Pan Film, Kodak | 2415 | Best source |
| 1.5-volt camera batteries | MS76 | " |
| Miniature lamps (osmometer) | G.E. 82 | " |
| Steril-Peel autoclave bags 5¼ × 10″ | | Hospital supply |
| Sodium heparin solution 5000 USP units | | Hospital pharmacy |
| Nunc freezer tubes | 366524 | Gibco |
| Ham's F-10 medium | 430-1200 | " |
| Dulbecco's PBS medium | 450-1300 | " |
| Calcium lactate | 4272 | Calbiochem/Behring |
| Benzyl penicillin G | PEN-NA | Sigma |
| Streptomycin sulfate | S6501 | " |
| Sodium bicarbonate | S8875 | " |
| Sharpie pens, blue | 13-5704-03 | Preiser |
| Propane burner | 10-8755-01 | " |
| Rogard prefilters | CDPRO1204 | Millipore |
| Super C carbon filters | CDFCO1204 | " |
| Ion exchange cartridges | CDMBO1202 | " |
| Millistak GS | MSGSO5CKZ | " |
| Total Count water tester | MT00 000 25 | " |
| Micro pH probe | MI-410 | Microelectrodes, Inc. |

# Morphology of Unfertilized and Fertilized Oocytes

## Meriella J. Hubbard and Leslie Weikert

### MATURATION OF THE OOCYTE

*Oogonia,* or primitive ova, are produced during fetal development by mitotic proliferation of primordial germ cells. After mitotic multiplication, the oogonia enter prophase of the first meiotic division and at this point they are primary oocytes. The primary oocyte consists of the ooplasm and a large prominent spherical nucleus or germinal vesicle. The nucleus of the primary oocyte enters the *dictyate,* or resting stage of the first meiotic prophase, and remains in the dictyate stage during growth of the oocyte and follicle during puberty and does not complete the first meiotic division until the follicle reaches maturity just prior to ovulation. Therefore, resumption of meiosis beyond the dictyate stage appears to depend on the ovulatory surge of luteinizing hormone. Shortly before ovulation, the oocyte undergoes the first meiotic division. The chromatin is divided equally between the daughter cells, but the division of the cytoplasm is extremely unequal. One of the daughter cells, termed the *secondary oocyte,* receives practically all of the cytoplasm of the mother cell; the other becomes the first polar body. In each, the chromosome number is reduced to a single set of 23 chromosomes.

At about this time, ovulation occurs and the nucleus of the secondary oocyte commences the second maturation division. The secondary oocyte is usually in metaphase II at ovulation and remains in this condition until fertilization.

### FERTILIZATION

At the time of ovulation or oocyte retrieval, the "mature" oocyte is generally surrounded by the zona pellucida, and this in turn is covered externally by a mass of granulosa cell layers called the *cumulus oophorus.* The granulosa cells of the cumulus oophorus directly in relation to the oocyte become radially arranged and form the *corona radiata* (Fig. 11-1). The mature or preovulatory oocyte is usually in metaphase II and is characterized by its association with an extruded first polar body (3).

In preparation for fertilization, the mature oocyte is incubated in vitro for 3–8 hours. After the predetermined incubation period is up, sperm are placed with the oocyte. The sperm penetrate and disperse the cumulus oophorus and corona radiata by the release of acrosomal enzymes. Proteolytic activity is also required for the sperm to penetrate the zona pellucida.

Therefore, fertilization is associated with the following events: (1) the contact of spermatozoa with the zona pellucida, penetration of one or more spermatozoa through the zona pellucida and the ooplasm, swelling of the sperm head, and extrusion of the second polar body in the perivitelline space; (2) the formation of the male and female pronuclei within the ooplasm; and (3) the beginning of the first mitotic division, or cleavage, of the zygote (2). In the case of human oocytes fertilized in vitro, pronuclei have been observed within 11 hours of insemination (1). In our laboratory, approximately 15–18 hours after insemination, the oocytes are examined and photographed for the occurrence of one or more of these parameters in order to assess fertilization (Figs. 11-2, 11-3, 11-4); however, the visualization of a second polar body or the existence of two pronuclei, or both, is not necessarily an indication of normal fertilization since the second polar body and the two pronuclei may be extruded and formed following parthenogenetic activation of the oocyte.

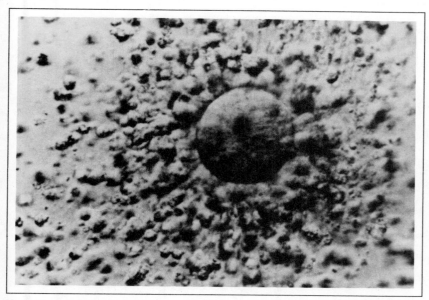

**Fig. 11-1.** Oocyte before fertilization, with the cumulus cells surrounding the zona pellucida.

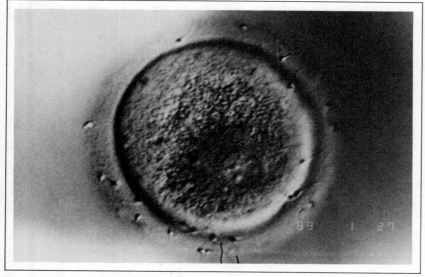

**Fig. 11-2.** Fertilized oocyte incubated 5½ hours prior to insemination. Two pronuclei found 15 hours post insemination (only one pronuclei visible).

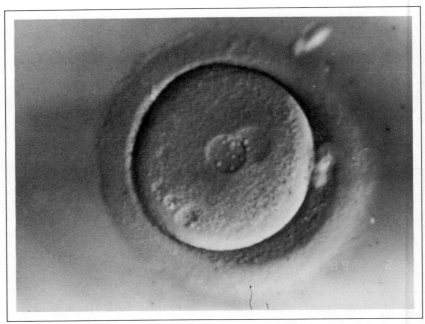

**Fig. 11-3.** Fertilized oocyte with two pronuclei and two polar bodies 15 hours post insemination. Oocyte incubated 5 hours prior to insemination.

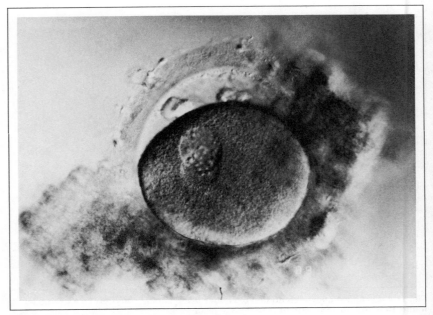

**Fig. 11-4.** Fertilized oocyte with two pronuclei.

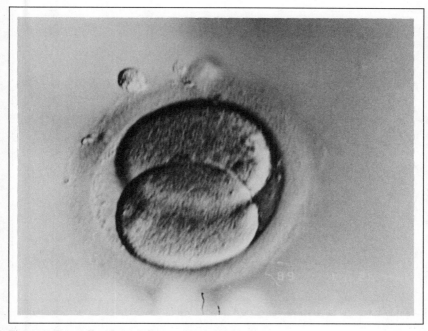

Fig. 11-5. Two-cell embryo 41 hours post insemination.

## CLEAVAGE

After fertilization is complete, the single-cell embryo divides and redivides many times without any increase in the overall size of its cytoplasm. This process of cellular division without growth is termed *cleavage* and it continues until blastocyst formation. During the early stages of cleavage, the embryonic cells are known as *blastomeres*. Normally cleaving two-cell concepti are observed any time after 22 hours post insemination, usually at around 24 hours, and may be seen until up to 44 hours post insemination (Fig. 11-5). Four-cell stages are routinely observed between 36 and 50 hours post insemination (Fig. 11-6), six to eight-cell stages after 48 hours (Fig. 11-7), and sixteen-cell stages after 68 hours (3). By the 16–32 cell stage, the cells are crowded together into a compact group within the zona pellucida and the embryo is now known as a *morula*. The divisions are not perfectly synchronized, so that three-, five-, and seven-cell stages may be found. All the divisions are mitotic; therefore, each cell of the embryo contains the diploid number of chromosomes (2n). It has been shown experimentally (in the mouse, rat, and rabbit) that a blastomere isolated from the mammalian two-cell organism is capable of forming a complete embryo, and in sheep and swine, normal embryos can develop from single blastomeres isolated at the four- to six-cell stage (2). In our laboratory, during the normal course of cleavage, each embryo is assessed morphologically to determine the number of blastomeres, their cytoplasmic conditions, and the presence of any blebs or fragments. Only four embryos are transferred back into the patient, and only those embryos that are judged to be developing "normally" are transferred 43–48 hours post insemination; however, it is recognized that "normality" based on morphologic interpretation is subjective and prone to error. If the oocyte has been

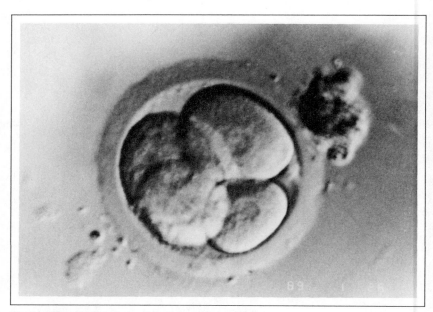

Fig. 11-6. Four-cell embryo 41 hours post insemination.

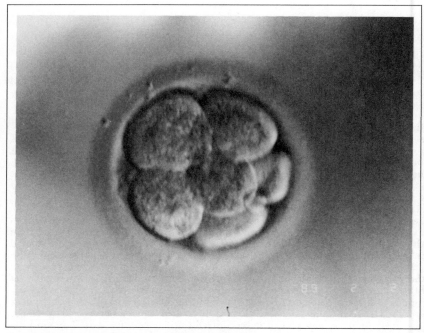

Fig. 11-7. Seven-cell embryo 44 hours post insemination.

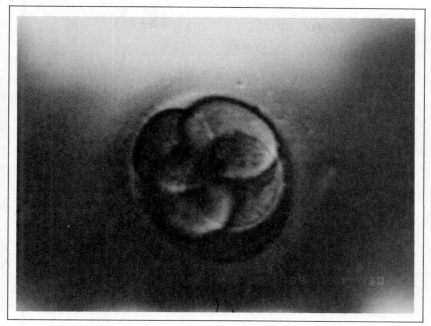

Fig. 11-8. Four-cell embryo post thaw. Embryo had been cryopreserved for 4 months.

fertilized normally and the blastomeres appear healthy, irrespective of their size or fragmentation, then the embryo is judged as normal and transferred. If the number of normal embryos exceeds four, then the excess embryos are frozen and thawed at a later date if implantation failed to occur after the first embryo transfer (Fig. 11-8).

## ABNORMAL OOCYTES

Several types of morphologic abnormalities such as a ruptured or fractured zona pellucida, empty zona (Figs. 11-9, 11-10), and atretic or degenerative ooplasm have been observed in unfertilized oocytes. These abnormalities may be due to inherent factors of the oocyte, environmental factors, or aging of the ovum.

## ABNORMAL FERTILIZATION

The complex process of fertilization is subject to several aberrations such as polyspermy, monospermic fertilization of an egg containing two female pronuclei, parthenogenesis, gynogenesis, and androgenesis.

Polyspermy occurs when extra sperm succeed in entering the ooplasm and thus multiple male pronuclei are formed (Fig. 11-11). Multiple pronuclei may also result from monospermic fertilization of binucleate ova. Two female pronuclei may develop from binucleate primary oocytes or as a result of failure to extrude the polar body at one of the maturation divisions.

Parthenogenesis, gynogenesis, and androgenesis occur when a single nucleus undergoes cleavage without syngamy. Specifically, in parthenogenesis the oocyte nucleus is activated in the absence of fertilization. In gynogenesis the oocyte is activated by a spermatozoa that then takes no further part in development. In androgenesis the nucleus of the oocyte fails to participate. The resulting

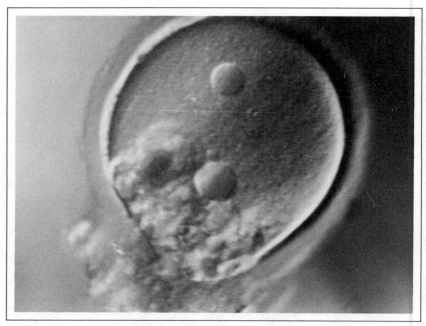

Fig. 11-9. Oocyte with fractured zona pellucida.

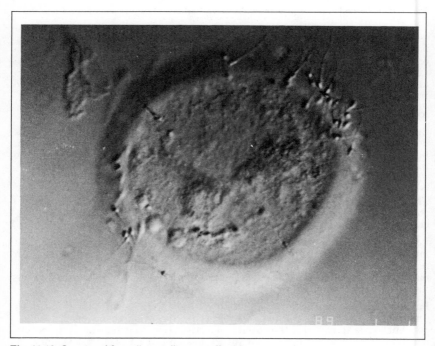

Fig. 11-10. Oocyte with an "empty" zona pellucida.

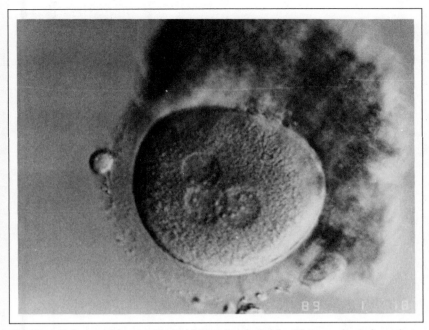

Fig. 11-11. Polyspermic oocyte that had been incubated for 5 hours prior to insemination. Three pronuclei photographed 15 hours post insemination.

embryos are destined to developmental failure and they generally fail to develop to birth.

Some of the causes of abnormal fertilization may be a result of aging of the gametes, poor culture conditions, elevation of environmental temperature, or exposure to certain toxic substances, or a combination of these.

## REFERENCES

1. Edwards, R. G. Fertilization and Cleavage In Vitro of Human Ova. In K. S. Moghissi and E. S. E. Hafez (eds.), *Biology of Mammalian Fertilization and Implantation.* Springfield IL: Thomas, 1972. Chap. 9, pp. 263–278.
2. O'Rahilly, R., and Muller, F. *Developmental Stages in Human Embryos, Including a Revision of Streeter's "Horizons" and a Survey of the Carnegie Collection.* Washington, DC: Carnegie Institution Washington Publication No. 637, 1987.
3. Veeck, L. L. *Atlas of the Human Oocyte and Early Conceptus.* Baltimore: Williams & Wilkins, 1986.

# Contemporary Procedures Associated with IVF-ET

# Gamete Intrafallopian Transfer: Current Perspectives

## Ricardo Azziz

Since the initial report of a birth following the reimplantation of a human embryo by Steptoe and Edwards in 1971 (44), in vitro fertilization and embryo transfer (IVF-ET) has resulted in fertility for many couples who otherwise would have been sterile; however, this technique has proved far from a panacea. The expense involved and the complexity of the laboratory setup preclude its ready accessibility. Furthermore, the actual birth rate appears to be less than 15% per retrieval (25), even at our most experienced centers (24,36). Various alternatives have been proposed to simplify and reduce the cost of IVF-ET. Bustillo and colleagues described the nonsurgical transfer of donor-fertilized ova (13). This procedure obviates the need for a laparoscopy/laparotomy, and the bulk of the in vitro laboratory. A fertile donor woman is artificially inseminated with sperm from the infertile patient's husband. Lavage of the donor's uterus is performed on the fifth day after the LH peak, with transvaginal recovery of the fertilized ovum. The embryo is then transferred into the infertile patient's uterus, which has been hormonally synchronized to the donor's cycle. Of 29 attempts, 12 ova were recovered and transferred, with two ongoing intrauterine pregnancies (13). Two complications were reported: an ectopic pregnancy in a recipient and a retained pregnancy in a donor that subsequently aborted spontaneously.

Another alternative to IVF-ET has been the transfer of laparoscopically recovered oocytes and washed sperm transvaginally into the uterus (15). After superovulation with clomiphene citrate, laparoscopic follicular aspiration is performed and the oocytes recovered and incubated for 6 hours. Sperm were then added to the incubation mixture for an additional hour, with subsequent intrauterine transfer of the gamete mixture. Of 31 patients, 14 (45%) demonstrated a positive human chorionic gonadotropin (hCG), although only two continuing pregnancies (6.4%) were reported. This technique greatly simplifies the laboratory requirements. Furthermore, oocyte retrieval performed transvaginally under sonography would obviate the need for abdominal puncture.

Forrler and colleagues reported the use of direct intraperitoneal insemination in cases of unexplained and cervical infertility (23). Ovulation induction was carried out using clomiphene citrate and human menopausal gonadotropin (hMG). At the time of ovulation, washed sperm were injected through the posterior vaginal fornix into the cul de sac, under sterile conditions. Three of ten patients demonstrated continuing pregnancies. In another report of the use of intraperitoneal insemination, Mason and colleagues noted that four of nine patients conceived with three continuing pregnancies (30); however, other investigators have not achieved the same success (19). The results of intraperitoneal insemination must be compared with the results of hMG superovulation combined with *intrauterine* insemination (IUI) in patients with unexplained infertility. Serhal and colleagues noted that the pregnancy rate per superovulated cycle was better if the insemination was performed by IUI (31.5%) than if IUI and intraperitoneal insemination were used together (20%), although the difference was not statistically significant (42). Another alternative to IVF-ET is the direct intrafallopian transfer of oocytes and sperm (51).

## EXPERIMENTAL BACKGROUND OF GAMETE INTRAFALLOPIAN TRANSFER

The experimental and theoretic background for gamete intrafallopian transfer (GIFT) centers on the ability of the fallopian tube to serve as the site of fertilization and sperm capacitation in humans. The transport of ova in the reproductive tract is characterized by their retention in the tubal ampulla for approximately 72 hours following ovulation (18), permitting fertilization to occur at this site (9,13). Furthermore, premature arrival of oocytes or embryos into the uterine cavity decreases the fertilization and implantation rate (2). Thus, the fallopian tube may coordinate the time of entry of the embryo into the uterine cavity in a more physiologic fashion than IVF-ET.

Sperm have been identified in the oviduct 5 minutes after deposition in the vagina of the human female (22). In spite of this extremely rapid transport system, the spermatozoa cannot fertilize the oocytes until full capacitation has occurred, which may take between 6–12 hours, depending on the species studied (12). In animals (boar and rabbit) (12,26), there appears to be synergism between the uterus and tube in producing sperm capacitation, although the factors provided by the fallopian tube appear to be of greater importance (12). Thus, intratubal insemination may lead to adequate sperm capacitation with subsequent oocyte fertilization.

Studies of GIFT in animal models have been few. Kreitmann and Hodgen reported pregnancies following low tubal-ovum transfers in monkeys (28). Bilateral resection and ligation of the ampullary region of the fallopian tubes were performed 1–2 cm from the utero-tubal junction, in rhesus and cynomologus monkeys. The follicle was aspirated laparoscopically and the identified oocyte injected into the lumen of the fallopian tube beyond its ligation. Pregnancy was detected in 5 of 31 attempts (16.1%). None of these pregnancies were ectopic, but unfortunately their ultimate outcome was not documented. Asch and colleagues performed GIFT on eight superovulated monkeys (7). Following hCG administration the preovulatory follicles were aspirated via laparotomy and GIFT was carried out. Pregnancy was confirmed biochemically in four of eight animals, three which subsequently aborted, with the fourth pregnancy continuing to term. With this scant but encouraging data, GIFT has been successfully utilized for the treatment of human infertility.

## CLINICAL DEVELOPMENT OF GIFT

In 1979 Schettles reported the intratubal transfer of freshly aspirated oocytes at the time of tubal reanastomosis (43). Cervical insemination was performed on the day prior to the operation. The patient was immediately pregnant and subsequently delivered a normal infant. In 1983 Tesarik and colleagues of Czechoslovakia reported two pregnancies in four women undergoing tubal microsurgery and tubal transfer of an oocyte/sperm mixture (45). One of these pregnancies continued to term.

Asch and colleagues first reported a pregnancy (5) and birth (6) following translaparoscopic GIFT in a patient with unexplained infertility. Initially Asch and colleagues utilized the laparoscope for gamete transfer, although they subsequently reported that they found it easier to perform the procedure by minilaparotomy (7). Currently the laparoscopic approach is favored.

## INDICATIONS AND PATIENT REQUIREMENTS FOR GIFT

GIFT has been utilized for the treatment of infertility for many assumed or proved abnormalities in the transfer of sufficient numbers of normal gametes into the fallopian tubes. With this broad application, GIFT has been used on patients with unexplained infertility, mild pelvic or tubal adhesions with and without endometriosis, cervical factor infertility with and without an immunologic component, failed conventional treatment of anovulatory disorders, failed artificial insemination by donor, or even premature ovarian failure (POF) utilizing donor oocytes. Couples with male factor infertility have also been candidates for GIFT. The specific results in each of these diagnostic subsets of patients will be described below.

The minimal patient prerequisites should be a complete infertility evaluation demonstrating at least one normal fallopian tube and a condition not amenable to less invasive treatment, as recently outlined by the American Fertility Society (3). Some investigators suggest the use of GIFT at the time of the initial diagnostic laparoscopy. Barad and colleagues achieved a 32% continuing pregnancy rate in 28 nulliparous patients who underwent GIFT performed at the time of their initial diagnostic procedure (11). All women with a history of pelvic infections, pelvic surgery, or positive findings on hysterosalpingography were excluded from this study. At this time, the use of GIFT with the initial diagnostic laparoscopy cannot be recommended, particularly with the advent of operative endoscopy. The presence of large superovulated ovaries may lead to suboptimal pelvic examination and deter from laparoscopic therapy for previously unrecognized pathology.

The arbitrary cutoff age has been 40 years in most programs. A recent report by Craft and colleagues (17) noted a 19.2% pregnancy rate among 193 women over the age of 40; however, almost 50% subsequently aborted for a final pregnancy success rate of 8%. The decision to accept patients into a GIFT program who are over the age of 40 years must be made on an individual basis.

The presence of at least one patent normal fallopian tube must be documented prior to undertaking GIFT. This information may be obtained from a previous laparoscopic examination; however, a concurrent hysterosalpingogram is highly recommended to rule out intraluminal disease or salpingitis isthmica nodosa. Tubal evaluation should have been performed within the year preceding GIFT. A history of previous ectopic pregnancies, with an otherwise normal-appearing pelvis, may be a relative contraindication to GIFT as it suggests intraluminal tubal disease.

Although male oligospermia is an indication for GIFT, a minimum number of motile sperm must be available. Usually at least 5 million sperm per ml must be present on semen analysis, with at least 30% motility. More important, a minimum of 1 million motile sperm must survive the sperm washing procedure in order to obtain enough sperm for transfer and potential IVF-ET of supernumerary oocytes. Asthenospermia should not be treated by GIFT. The exact sperm number requirements will be discussed below.

An adequate response to superovulatory medications is obviously needed in order to produce a sufficient number of oocytes. Although GIFT has been performed with single oocytes, the success rates are significantly less than if four or more are transferred. In rare circumstances (premature ovarian failure), GIFT has been performed using donor oocytes.

## CHOOSING BETWEEN GIFT AND IVF-ET

For couples who have completed their infertility evaluation and have not responded to conventional treatment, the so-called assisted reproductive technologies are available. Women who demonstrate at least one apparently normal fallopian tube may be candidates for both IVF-ET and GIFT. Deciding which technique to utilize must be individualized for each patient.

The theoretic advantages of GIFT over IVF include (1) fertilization occurs at its natural site, i.e., the tubal ampulla, (2) the gametes are minimally exposed to the extracorporal environment, (3) the embryos are prevented from prematurely entering into the endometrial cavity, and (4) early embryo development does not occur in an artificial environment, which may be retarded in an in vitro setting.

Alternatively, IVF-ET has certain advantages over GIFT including (1) fertilization of the oocyte is clearly documented, whereas no such information is obtained with GIFT unless a pregnancy intervenes, (2) with the advent of transvaginal sonography and follicle aspiration, the degree of trauma and anesthetic risk to the patient is greatly minimized in comparison to the need for laparoscopy/laparotomy with GIFT, and (3) during GIFT the abdomen must be insufflated, usually exposing the oocytes to an environment high in carbon dioxide, which may be detrimental to the subsequent development (31).

Although the theoretic advantages of GIFT suggest a higher success rate over IVF-ET, supportive data are scant. With the first report of the United States IVF-ET registry, the clinical pregnancy rate for GIFT was 23.2% per treatment cycle for 1986, and 16.9% per transfer cycle for IVF-ET (36). This report was a collection of the results of many different clinics and did not control for diagnosis, patient selection, and many other factors affecting the success rates. Yovich, Yovich, and Eidrisinghe reported the relative chances of pregnancy following IVF-ET or GIFT in a 7-month study in their medical center. The pregnancy rate per transfer was 12.5% for IVF-ET, significantly lower than that for GIFT (35.9%) (51).

In spite of these encouraging data, a recent randomized controlled trial between GIFT and IVF-ET showed no significant differences in the pregnancy rates of couples presenting with idiopathic or male infertility. Leeton and colleagues randomized 86 couples with unexplained infertility and 14 couples with male infertility problems (29). If the initially selected treatment modality failed, the patients were treated with the alternative method at their next attempt. The pregnancy success for couples with unexplained infertility was 19% with GIFT and 20% for IVF-ET. For male factor infertility it was 33 and 28.5%, respectively. Although the study did not demonstrate that GIFT was superior to IVF-ET in these couples, it should be noted that the overall success rate of GIFT was significantly lower than has been reported by most other investigators. Furthermore, the pregnancy rate was higher for male infertility patients than for those with idiopathic infertility, which also does not agree with other centers' results. This may suggest that these investigators did not have a representative patient population. Further investigations are required before GIFT is established as more successful than IVF-ET for couples in which the woman has at least one normal fallopian tube and the man sufficient sperm numbers.

It has been suggested that GIFT is at least 25–30% less expensive than IVF-ET because of the reduction in laboratory needs. Such a differential in cost does not exist today because IVF-ET can usually be performed by transvaginal follicle aspiration, obviating the need for laparoscopy. Thus, the differential in laboratory costs is offset by the operative expenses of endoscopy with GIFT. The cost for either procedure ranges from $3000.00–6000.00 per cycle, depending on the center.

## CURRENT CLINICAL RESULTS OF GIFT

The reported biochemical pregnancy rate per laparoscopic GIFT attempt ranges from 21–44% (10,17,24,27,29,35,38,50) with an average of 26%. The clinical pregnancy rate per GIFT attempt ranges from 18–32% (Table 12-1) in this same series of reports, with an average of 21%. Clinical pregnancies are defined somewhat differently in each of these studies. As previously mentioned, age is an important factor affecting pregnancy rates following GIFT. Craft and colleagues noted that 19.2% of women over the age of 40 became pregnant provided *all* their oocytes were transformed, compared to 35% for women between ages 30–34 years (17). Unfortunately, almost half of the pregnancies in women over 40 subsequently aborted.

The degree of experience with the GIFT appears to influence pregnancy rates. From the United States IVF-ET registry, a clinical pregnancy rate of 5.4% was noted for the first 56 GIFT cycles recorded in 1985. The total number of cycles increased ninefold to 419 in 1986, and with this increased experience the pregnancy rate rose to 23.2% per treatment cycle (36). At the Arizona Center for Fertility Studies, Nemiro and McGauhey reported a 20% pregnancy rate per

**Table 12-1. Success rate of GIFT for all couples through 1988**

| Author, yr | Reference | Transfers | Total pregnancies per transfer (%) | Total clinical pregnancies per transfer (%) |
|---|---|---|---|---|
| Asch et al., 1986 | 10 | 100 | 28 | 18 |
| Guastella et al., 1986 | 24 | 44 | 39 | 32 |
| IVF-ET Registry, 1986 | 26 | 416 | 28 | 19 |
| Nemiro and McGaughey, 1986 | 38 | 60 | 30 | 20 |
| Leeton et al., 1987 | 29 | 43 | 21 | — |
| McGaughey and Nemiro, 1987 | 35 | 61 | 44 | 29 |
| Molloy et al., 1987 | 37 | 71 | 32 | 27 |
| Craft et al., 1988 | 17 | 1071 | 34 | 25 |
| Khan et al., 1988 | 27 | 305 | 28 | 19 |
| Yovich et al., 1988* | 50 | 207 | 24 | 21 |
| Overall | | 2378 | 26 | 21 |

*Reported only normospermic couples.

Table 12-2. Number of first-trimester fetuses following GIFT: relation to number of oocytes transferred

| No. of oocytes transferred | No. of pregnancies | Pregnancies (%) | | |
|---|---|---|---|---|
| | | One fetus | Two fetuses | ≥ Three fetuses |
| 1–2 | 16 | 94 | 6 | — |
| 3–4 | 65 | 80 | 15 | 5 |
| 5–6 | 118 | 77 | 14 | 7 |
| 7–8 | 104 | 61 | 28 | 12 |
| 9–10 | 41 | 56 | 29 | 15 |

Source: Modified from I. Craft et al. Analysis of 1071 GIFT procedures--the case for a flexible approach to treatment. *Lancet* 1(8594):1094, 1988.

Table 12-3. Pregnancy success of GIFT: relation to the number of oocytes transferred

| No. of oocytes transferred | No. of patients | Pregnancies (%) |
|---|---|---|
| 1–2 | 115 | 14 |
| 3–4 | 263 | 25 |
| 5–6 | 310 | 38 |
| 7–8 | 243 | 43 |
| 9–10 | 108 | 38 |

Source: Modified from I Craft et al. Analysis of 1071 GIFT procedures—the case for a flexible approach to treatment. *Lancet* 1(8594):1094, 1988.

laparoscopy in their first 60 such attempts (38). Subsequently, in their second series of 61 laparoscopies, they reported a 29% pregnancy rate (35). Their cancellation rate per cycle was approximately the same (56 and 57%, respectively). These data strongly suggest that increasing clinical experience with this method of assisted reproduction will lead to improved results.

## Multiple Gestations versus Pregnancy Success

The incidence of multiple gestations has been a constant preoccupation with GIFT and IVF-ET since both techniques transfer a large number of oocytes/embryos. The incidence of multiple gestations ranges from 17–55% of all GIFT clinical pregnancies (17,29,35,37,38,50). Most of the multiple gestations occur with the placement of four or more oocytes (17,38,50). Craft and colleagues reported that the multiple pregnancy rate was approximately 40% with the placement of seven or more oocytes and remained relatively stable throughout (17) (Table 12-2).

Although the number of multiple gestations appears to be related to the number of oocytes transferred, the pregnancy rate of GIFT also depends on the number of oocytes transferred. In the same report by Craft and colleagues (17), the pregnancy rate was approximately 40% for patients receiving five or more oocytes compared to 14% if only one or two oocytes was transferred (Table 12-3). The relationship of oocytes transferred and pregnancy rate has been confirmed by others (37,38,51).

## Ectopic Pregnancies

Ectopic pregnancy rates following GIFT range from 0–8% with an average of 4% of all pregnancies (2,10,17,24,35,37,38,50). This does not appear to be much higher than the ectopic rate associated with IVF-ET alone (36). It is not known whether the incidence of ectopic pregnancies following GIFT is further increased in patients with peritubal adhesions and previous ectopics. Bilateral ectopic pregnancies (39) and combined intra-abdominal/intrauterine pregnancies have been reported following GIFT (1).

## Spontaneous Abortions and Abnormal Births

The spontaneous abortion rate ranges from 22–35% in the various reports (17,27,36) and appears to be comparable to that of IVF-ET (36). The incidence of spontaneous abortion after GIFT rises dramatically after age 40 with almost half of the clinical pregnancies ending in miscarriage (17). The number of oocytes transferred does not appear to affect the miscarriage rate.

The incidence of abnormal births and congenital anomalies with GIFT is not known. There is no reason to believe that their obstetric outcome should be any different from that obtained with IVF-ET or with normal gestations, taking into consideration the complications associated with multiple gestations. Reporting on 125 consecutive pregnancies conceived by IVF-ET in Norfolk, Andrews and colleagues noted that the complications of pregnancy were similar to those of comparable populations with the exception of eight deliveries under 36 weeks. Two of these were twin pregnancies and one triplet (4).

## GIFT Therapy of Unexplained Infertility

GIFT has been used most often in couples with idiopathic infertility in which no obvious tubal defect is noted. In a review of the literature, of 280 GIFT procedures performed in patients with unexplained infertility, 87 patients became pregnant for an average success rate of 31% (24,27,35,37,38,50). In order to determine whether this success rate is an improvement over currently available and less invasive methods, the outcome of ovulation induction with or without IUI in couples with unexplained infertility should be evaluated. Yovich and Matson noted that 15 of 183 (8%) couples with unexplained infertility achieved pregnancy after IUI and selective ovulation induction, compared to 7 of 25 (28%) couples undergoing GIFT for the same diagnosis. This study was not randomized or controlled (48). Utilizing hMG superovulation and IUI in couples with unexplained infertility, Serhal and colleagues reported that 26.4% (9 of 34) of the treatment cycles led to pregnancy (42). Dodson and colleagues reported an overall pregnancy rate of 16% per cycle with the use of IUI and hMG superovulation in 148 couples with idiopathic infertility (21). In this cumulative study, the pregnancy rate was 35% although no pregnancies occurred after the second treatment cycle. It would appear that GIFT should be reserved for couples with unexplained infertility who do not achieve pregnancy following an adequate trial of hMG superovulation and IUI.

## GIFT for the Treatment of Male Factor Infertility

There has been much controversy as to the use of GIFT for couples in which the male demonstrates a decreased number of motile sperm. Of 32 treatment cycles in 17 couples with oligospermia, a 15% clinical success rate was reported by Nemiro and McGaughey (38). These investigators also noted a significant difference in the mean seminal parameters between pregnant and nonpregnant patients. The mean sperm count was 139 million per ml in patients achieving pregnancy compared to 176 million per ml in nonpregnant women; however, motility did not vary significantly, 56 versus 52%, respectively. Interestingly, the number of motile sperm transferred was higher in nonpregnant than pregnant cycles. Although the motility of the sperm used for insemination appeared to be statistically higher in cycles achieving pregnancy, the difference was minimal.

Matson and associates reported that of 32 oligospermic couples ($< 12 \times 10^6$ *motile* sperm per ml), no pregnancies were conceived when 100,000 sperm were transferred per tube (32,34); however, if a maximum number of motile sperm were placed in the tubes, 6 of 21 cycles (29%) resulted in pregnancy. No conceptions were recorded if less than 325,000 sperm per tube were used. The effect of sperm number appears to be independent of the number of oocytes transferred. In a simultaneously published study from the same clinic, a 21% pregnancy rate was reported for normospermic couples (50). These data suggested that the sperm of oligospermic males have a reduced fertility potential that can be overcome by increasing the number of motile sperm transferred.

Alternatively, Leeton and colleagues (29) utilized only 100,000 sperm per two oocytes transferred in 37 GIFT cycles in oligospermic couples (< 20 million *total* sperm per ml, with motility > 40%, and normal forms (< 40%), and reported a 33% pregnancy rate. In another study, Khan and colleagues were not able to demonstrate a decreased pregnancy success rate with as little as 5000 sperm transferred per three oocytes (only one tube was cannulated), in patients with either idiopathic or andrologic infertility (27). With 2500 sperm per three oocytes, a 34% pregnancy rate was still achieved in patients with unexplained infertility, although the success rate dropped to 6% (1 of 16) of cycles in male factor couples. Moreover, utilizing 100,000 sperm, these investigators noted a slightly decreased success rate, 29 and 12%, respectively, for idiopathic and male infertility patients.

In comparing IVF-ET and GIFT for the treatment of oligospermia, Leeton and colleagues were not able to demonstrate a significant difference in pregnancy rates in their prospective randomized trial (29). As previously noted, this study had an unusually high success rate for male infertility suggesting a possible bias in patient selection.

Comparing GIFT to IUI for the treatment of oligospermia, Yovich and Matson have reported an 8% pregnancy rate following the use of IUI and selective ovulation induction in 66 couples with oligospermia, compared to a 29% success rate in 21 couples treated with GIFT for the same diagnosis (48). This suggests that GIFT has an improved success rate over IUI for the treatment of oligospermic infertility. Furthermore, these investigators were not able to achieve any pregnancies in couples with asthenospermia.

Although these studies suggest that GIFT is an appropriate treatment for oligospermic infertility, it is not clear whether increasing the number of motile sperm transferred per oocyte leads to an increase or decrease in pregnancy rates. Furthermore, in IVF-ET polyspermic fertilization has been related to the total number of sperm used per oocyte (46). Insemination of oocytes with relatively low sperm concentrations ($0.5-0.8 \times 10^6$ sperm per oocyte) resulted in a polyspermic rate of 7%. Higher sperm concentrations of $1 \times 10^6$ and $1.5 \times 10^6$ sperm per oocyte led to a polyploidy rate of 13 and 18%, respectively. In spite of this in vitro data, Khan and colleagues did not observe a decrease in the spontaneous abortion rate when reducing the number of sperm transferred at the time of GIFT (27). Further studies are required in this area.

### GIFT for Other Causes of Infertility

In a review of the literature, 16 of 50 (32%) of patients with pelvic adhesions, 13 of 44 (29%) women with mild peritubular adhesions, 20 of 98 (20%) of endometriosis, and 11 of 53 (21%) of couples with cervical infertility achieved pregnancy using GIFT (24,27,35,37,38,50). Recently Asch and colleagues reported the treatment of eight patients with POF with GIFT using donated oocytes (8). These oocytes were obtained from patients in their GIFT program after transfer. Six clinical pregnancies were achieved in eight cycles (75%). Prior to transfer of the donated oocytes, hormonal synchronization between donor and recipient was performed. If the reported pregnancy rate for POF is confirmed, GIFT could become a very promising treatment for this frustrating disorder.

## GIFT OUTSIDE THE IVF LABORATORY?

As the use of GIFT becomes widespread, its indications broaden and the technique is simplified. Pavlou and Pampiglione reported a GIFT pregnancy utilizing a portable laboratory (40). Notwithstanding, various investigators cautioned against performing GIFT without proper IVF-ET support (16,32). The reasons are multiple: (1) GIFT may not be able to be performed because of unexpected fallopian tube damage or other technical difficulties, (2) the technical expertise required for oocyte handling and appropriate culture media are usually present in clinics who also have ongoing IVF-ET, (3) without IVF-ET and cryopreservation, the disposal of excess oocytes becomes an ethical and psychological problem, and (4) a cycle of GIFT not resulting in pregnancy provides no information on the fecundability of the couple. The IVF of supernumerary oocytes and subsequent embryo cryopreservation may have significant diagnostic and therapeutic value. The American Fertility Society states that a gamete laboratory and personnel meeting the standards of an IVF program are part of the minimal requirements for a GIFT program (3).

It is not clear to what extent the IVF of supernumerary oocytes from a GIFT cycle is useful for assessing a couple's fecundability and the future success rate of the procedure (41). Quigley and colleagues reported on the use of a combined IVF/GIFT procedure. All 16 couples had at least *two* oocytes used for GIFT and *two* oocytes inseminated in vitro. Only one couple (6.25%) achieved a clinical pregnancy in this series. These investigators noted that 50% of these couples also had no oocytes fertilized in vitro. These investigators suggested that in all couples in which fecundability has not previously been documented, GIFT should be performed along with IVF. It is important to note that in this study, the overall success rate of GIFT was extremely low, and that 4 of 16 couples were transferred only two oocytes. Alternatively, Matson and colleagues questioned the value of the failure of supernumerary oocytes after GIFT to fertilize in vitro (33). In their study of 42 couples, *four* oocytes were always replaced in the fallopian tubes. The remaining oocytes were then inseminated in vitro. Their overall GIFT pregnancy rate was 40% in normospermic couples. These authors did not find a correlation between the IVF rate and the GIFT pregnancy success. It should be noted that these studies present conflicting information that may be related to their significantly different criteria for oocyte selection and transfer. In the study by Quigley and colleagues, the number of oocytes was divided equally between those kept for IVF and those transferred into the fallopian tube (41). Alternatively, Matson and colleagues always attempted to transfer *at least* four oocytes into the fallopian tube, leaving 69.2% of the couples with only one oocyte for IVF (33). These data taken together suggest that the predictive value of IVF of low numbers of preselected oocytes is limited; however, the IVF of greater numbers of supernumerary mature and normal-appearing oocytes may be therapeutically and diagnostically valuable.

## TECHNIQUE OF GAMETE INTRAFALLOPIAN TRANSFER

GIFT requires superovulation with the production of a large number of follicles containing mature oocytes. Superovulation is followed by follicle aspiration, microscopic examination, and oocyte selection. The oocytes are then loaded into a catheter together with previously washed sperm. The gametes are finally transferred into the ampullary region of the fallopian tube(s) laparoscopically.

### Ovulation Induction

Ovulation induction has been carried out with a number of agents including clomiphene only, clomiphene and hMG, and hMG only. No consistent difference in pregnancy rates has been reported, although fewer mature oocytes are recovered with clomiphene alone, a factor that has been associated with a reduced success rate. Overall, the mode of ovulation induction, its drawbacks, and risks are very similar to those of IVF-ET (see Chap. 7 and 8). McGaughey and Nemiro reported on the association of estradiol ($E_2$) levels during ovulation induction and the outcome of GIFT (35). In 59 transfers the total $E_2$ and the $E_2$ levels per follicle were higher for pregnant than for nonpregnant women. Although the mean number of preovulatory oocytes obtained in these two groups of patients did not differ, the mean number of mature oocytes recovered was significantly higher if pregnancy was achieved. Interestingly, more than half of the pregnancies with very high preovulatory levels of serum $E_2$ ($2683 \pm 20$ pg/ml) were only biochemical without subsequent evidence of clinical pregnancy. This study suggests that a maximum incidence of clinical pregnancies with GIFT occurs with serum $E_2$ levels of between 300 and 500 pg/ml per follicle, with higher and lower values associated with a decreased success (35). High estrogen levels resulting in a greater incidence of biochemical pregnancies have not been observed previously in IVF-ET cycles. It is possible that abnormally high $E_2$ levels may interfere with early embryo development in vivo or with embryo implantation.

## Oocyte Retrieval

Follicular aspiration and oocyte retrieval are performed 34–36 hours following the administration of hCG as outlined for IVF-ET in Chap. 8. If clomiphene was used exclusively, the retrieval is performed 24–48 hours after the spontaneous urinary LH surge. Oocyte retrieval is usually performed laparoscopically, with few exceptions, as detailed for IVF-ET. In selected patients with extensive cul de sac and periovarian adhesions, it may be easier to first perform transvaginal follicular aspiration, followed by laparoscopy for intrafallopian gamete transfer.

## Sperm Preparation

Sperm preparation for GIFT must increase the number of motile sperm while reducing the presence of irritants or infectious organisms. Semen is collected by masturbation, after 3 days of abstinence, approximately 2 hours before the oocyte retrieval. Following liquefaction a small aliquot is taken for microscopic semen analysis. If the husband has normal seminal parameters, approximately 1 ml of liquified semen is used; however, in oligospermic couples the entire seminal volume is used. For the first wash the semen aliquot is thoroughly mixed with two volumes of Ham's F-10 supplemented with 7.5% maternal serum and penicillin 12,000 units 100 per ml (modified Ham's F-10 media). The specimen is then centrifuged at 400 g (gravity) for 15 minutes. The supernatant is discarded and the sperm pellet is resuspended in 1 ml of modified Ham's F-10 media, thoroughly mixed and recentrifuged. After again discarding the supernatant, 0.5 ml of modified Ham's F-10 media is layered carefully over the sperm pellet. After 60–90 minutes during which the motile sperm "swim-up" into the overlying media, the supernatant is carefully aspirated and saved. A small amount of this fluid containing the motile sperm is analyzed microscopically and the total volume of the sample adjusted with modified Ham's F-10 media to give a sperm concentration of approximately 4 million per ml. This sperm preparation is maintained in a gas incubator (5% carbon dioxide 37°C) or gased (with 5% carbon dioxide, 5% oxygen, and 9% nitrogen) and left at room temperature until used.

## Oocyte Preparation

Once the oocytes have been retrieved, they are graded for maturity by evaluating the expansion of the cumulus and corona radiata (per Norfolk classification). Each oocyte is placed in individual culture dishes with 100 µl of modified Ham's F-10 media. Four to six of the most mature oocytes are than selected for subsequent intrafallopian transfer. The exact number of oocytes used will depend on the patient's age, the appearance of the oocytes, and the couple's choice after discussion of the risk of multiple pregnancies versus the overall pregnancy success rate.

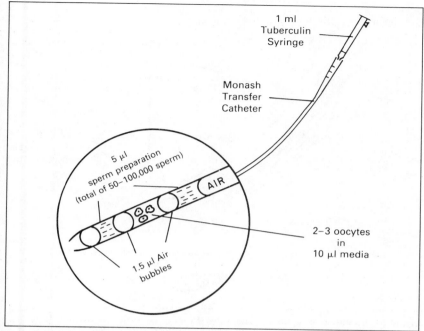

**Fig. 12-1. Loading of the gametes for the GIFT procedure.**

## Gamete Loading

A number of catheters have been used for GIFT, including a 24-in. 16-gauge Deseret Intracath (Deseret Co., Sandy, UT No. 3132) and a stirrable GIFT catheter by Cook ob/gyn (Cook, Inc.) (14). We prefer to use the Monash embryo transfer catheter, which is initially flushed 2–3 times with modified Ham's F-10 media. A 1-ml tuberculin syringe is attached to the end of the catheter and the gametes are loaded. Filling the catheter should not be started until the surgeon has cannulated the tube length, reducing the time the embryos are allowed to inevitably cool.

Initially 5 μl of sperm preparation containing approximately 50,000 sperm is aspirated. This is followed by a 1.5-μl air bubble and then by 10 μl of media containing two to three oocytes. Following the oocytes, another 1.5-μl air bubble is aspirated. Now 5 μl of sperm preparation is taken up into the catheter and finally another 1.5-μl air bubble is aspirated (Fig. 12-1). The procedure is repeated for each tube transferred. The exact purpose of the air bubbles is not clear although they may contribute to maintaining the gamete within the transfer catheter by increased capillary action.

As discussed previously, a higher number of sperm may be transferred for patients with oligospermic infertility, and a higher number of oocytes may be used in patients over the age of 40.

## Gamete Intrafallopian Transfer

Although some authors have utilized a minilaparotomy for tubal cannulation, most transfers today are performed by laparoscopy. After the laparoscope is

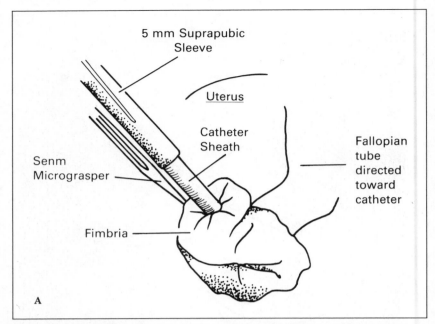

**Fig. 12-2A. Cannulation of the fallopian tube. (From R. H. Asch et al. Gamete intra-fallopian transfer (GIFT): A new treatment for infertility. *Int. J. Fertil.* 30:41, 1985. With permission.)**

inserted, a small suprapubic incision is performed through which the grasping instrument is placed. A second smaller 3-mm incision is made approximately 4 cm below the umbilicus through which the Monash transfer catheter and sheath are placed. At this time, peritubular lysis of adhesions is performed if necessary. Although many instruments for tubal grasping have been reported, this author prefers the Semm micrograsper (Wisap Co., UI.S.A. No. 7678-F). The antimesenteric portion of the tube is gently grasped behind the origin of the fimbria. Although some surgeons suggest putting the entire tube on stretch for easy cannulation, this author finds that principally directing the tubal ostia toward the transfer catheter greatly facilitates cannulation. In this manner the tube drapes down and is not on full stretch (Fig. 12-2A, B). Once the fimbria are cannulated, the tube can then be stretched over the transfer catheter. It is easier to catheterize the tubal ostia immediately below the grasping forceps by first probing with an empty transfer catheter extended beyond the sheath and not with the sheath proper. Once the tube is cannulated, the empty transfer catheter is advanced into the ampullary isthmic junction. Using the marking on the proximal part of the transfer catheter, the tip is advanced at least 2 cm beyond its sheath. It is extremely important to verify adequate placement of the catheter within the tube since the catheter may curl downward through the fimbria and into the cul de sac, appearing to have cannulated the ampulla.

A loaded transfer catheter is now brought into the operating room in a sterile fashion on a Mayo tray and delivered to the surgeon. The cannulating empty GIFT catheter is removed, leaving the sheath within the tubal ampulla. The surgeon then passes the loaded GIFT catheter through the sheath into its proper position within the tube (Fig. 12-3). The catheter contents are then carefully ejected, and, after approximately 15 seconds, the entire catheter and sheath are

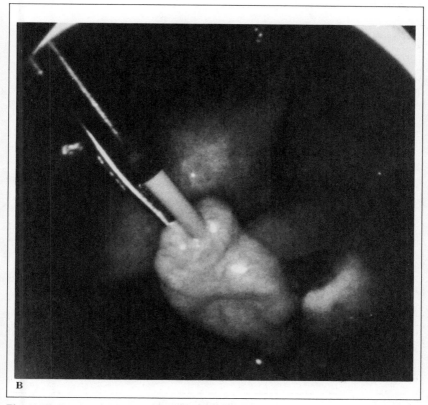

**Fig. 12-2B. Laparoscopic view of tubal cannulation.**

removed with a slight shaking motion. It is important to maintain the transfer catheter beyond the sheath at all times in order to avoid injecting the gametes into the sheath and subsequently withdrawing them.

The unloaded GIFT catheter is removed and returned to the laboratory. The catheter is flushed with a small volume of modified Ham's F-10 media and the washings examined under the microscope to determine whether any oocytes were retained. An identical procedure is performed on the opposite fallopian tube if available. The cannulation and transfer of gametes into each fallopian tube should take no more than 10 minutes. After the gamete tubal transfers are completed, the tubes are left undisturbed and the pelvis is not lavaged.

### Luteal Support and Follow-up

Progesterone supplementation is begun 3 days after the tubal transfer as out-lined for IVF-ET. A serum β-hCG is obtained 12–14 days after gamete transfer.

## FUTURE IMPROVEMENTS IN GAMETE TUBAL TRANSFER

A major disadvantage of GIFT is that fertilization cannot be verified unless a pregnancy ensues. This information is particularly important in couples with severe oligospermia or other male infertility problems. Furthermore, the absence of oocyte fertilization may suggest a basic defect in either sperm or ova function,

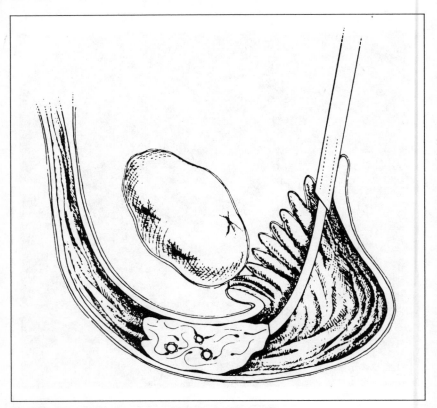

**Fig. 12-3. Placement of gametes within the tubal ampulla.**

thus having significant diagnostic value. In order to overcome some of these disadvantages, the technique of pronuclear stage tubal transfer (PROST) or zygote intrafallopian transfer was developed. In this system the oocytes are retrieved as they are for IVF-ET, preferably transvaginally, and subsequently inseminated. Once fertilization is confirmed by the presence of two pronuclei within the oocytes, three to four zygotes are transferred into the fallopian tubes laparoscopically (usually the day after oocyte retrieval). The first pregnancy with this technique was reported by Devroey and colleagues (20). Yovich and colleagues subsequently reported 30 pregnancies of 81 transfers (37%), compared to a 36% pregnancy rate per GIFT transfer (49). In this study, PROST was usually reserved for couples with infertility due to oligospermia or asthenospermia, when either partner demonstrated significant levels of antispermatozoal antibodies, or when significant levels of any circulating antibody subtype were observed in the female partner (23). PROST may be a useful alternative in select couples with unproved fecundability.

The need for laparoscopic tubal cannulation during GIFT is a major deterrent to its widespread and repeated use, particularly since IVF-ET today utilizes transvaginal follicle aspiration in the majority of patients. Transvaginal retrograde cannulation of the fallopian tubes, either under ultrasonic or hysteroscopic guidance would greatly increase the utility of GIFT. Wurfel and colleagues recently reported a pregnancy following intratubal gamete transfer under hysteroscopic guidance (47). Further work in this area will certainly lead to a reduction in the cost of GIFT and its increased availability.

## REFERENCES

1. Abdalla, H. I., et al. Combined intraabdominal and intrauterine pregnancies after gamete intrafallopian transfer. *Lancet* 2:1153, 1986.
2. Adams, C. E. Consequences of accelerated ovum transport, including a re-evaluation of Estes' operation. *J. Reprod. Fertil.* 55:239, 1979.
3. American Fertility Society. Minimal standards for gamete intrafallopian transfer (GIFT). *Fertil. Steril.* 50:20, 1988.
4. Andrews, M. C., et al. An analysis of the obstetric outcome of 125 consecutive pregnancies conceived in vitro and resulting in 100 deliveries. *Am. J. Obstet. Gynecol.* 154:858, 1986.
5. Asch, R. H., et al. Pregnancy after translaparoscopic gamete intrafallopian transfer. *Lancet* 2:1034, 1984.
6. Asch, R. H., et al. Birth following gamete intrafallopian transfer. *Lancet* 2:163, 1985.
7. Asch, R. H., et al. Gamete intrafallopian transfer (GIFT): Use of minilaparotomy and an individualized regimen of induction of follicular development. *Acta Eur. Fertil.* 17:187, 1986.
8. Asch, R. H., et al. Oocyte donation and gamete intrafallopian transfer in premature ovarian failure. *Fertil. Steril.* 49:263, 1988.
9. Austin, C. R., and Bishop, M. W. H. Fertilization in mammals. *Biol. Rev.* 32:296, 1957.
10. Balmaceda, J. P., et al. Results in 100 consecutive cases of infertility treated with gamete intrafallopian transfer (GIFT). American Fertility Society abstracts, P-074, 1986.
11. Barad, D. H., et al. Gamete intrafallopian tube transfer (GIFT): Making laparoscopy more than "diagnostic". *Fertil. Steril.* 50:928, 1988.
12. Bedford, J. M. Limitations of the uterus in the development of the fertilizing ability (capacitation) of spermatozoa. *J. Reprod. Fertil. [Suppl.]* 8:19, 1969.
13. Bustillo, M., et al. Nonsurgical ovum transfer as a treatment in infertile women. *J.A.M.A.* 251:1171, 1984.
14. Confino, E., Friberg, J., and Gleicher, N. New stirrable catheter for gamete intrafallopian tube transfer (GIFT). *Fertil. Steril.* 46:1147, 1986.
15. Craft, I., et al. Human pregnancy following oocyte and sperm transfer to the uterus. *Lancet* 1:1031, 1982.
16. Craft, I., et al. Limitations of GIFT. *Lancet* 1:183, 1988.
17. Craft, I., et al. Analysis of 1,071 GIFT procedures—the case for a flexible approach to treatment. *Lancet* 1:1094, 1988.
18. Croxatto, H. B., et al. Studies on the duration of egg transport by the human oviduct. II. Ovum location at various intervals following luteinizing hormone peak. *Am. J. Obstet. Gynecol.* 132:629, 1978.
19. Curson, R., and Parsons, J. Disappointing results with direct intraperitoneal insemination. *Lancet* 1:112, 1987.
20. Devroey, P., et al. Pregnancy after translaparoscopic zygote intrafallopian transfer in a patient with sperm antibodies. *Lancet* 1:1329, 1986.
21. Dodson, W. C., et al. Superovulation with intrauterine insemination in the treatment of infertility: A possible alternative to gamete intrafallopian transfer and in vitro fertilization. *Fertil. Steril.* 48:441, 1987.
22. Fordney-Settlage, D. S., Motoshima, M., and Tredway, D. R. Sperm transport from the external cervical os to the fallopian tubes in women: A time and quantitation study. *Fertil. Steril.* 24:655, 1973.
23. Forrler, A., et al. Direct intraperitoneal insemination in unexplained and cervical infertility. *Lancet* 2:916, 1986.
24. Guastella, G., et al. Gamete intrafallopian transfer in the treatment of infertility: The first series at the University of Palermo. *Fertil. Steril.* 46:417, 1986.

25. Guzick, D. S., Wilkes, C., and Jones, H. W., Jr. Cumulative pregnancy rates for in vitro fertilization. *Fertil. Steril.* 46:663, 1986.
26. Hunter, R. H. F. and Hall, J. P. Capacitation of boar spermatozoa: Synergism between uterine and tubal environments. *J. Exp. Zool.* 188:203, 1974.
27. Khan, I., et al. Success rate in gamete intrafallopian transfer using low and high concentrations of washed spermatozoa. *Fertil. Steril.* 50:922, 1988.
28. Kreitmann, O., and Hodgen, G. D. Low tubal ovum transfer: An alternative to in vitro fertilization. *Fertil. Steril.* 34:375, 1980.
29. Leeton, J., et al. A controlled study between the use of gamete intrafallopian transfer (GIFT) and in vitro fertilization and embryo transfer in the management of idiopathic and male infertility. *Fertil. Steril.* 48:605, 1987.
30. Mason, B., et al. Ultrasound guided peritoneal oocyte and sperm transfer (POST). *Lancet* 1:386, 1987.
31. Mastroyannia, C., et al. The effect of a carbon dioxide pneumoperitoneum on rabbit follicular oocytes and early embryonic development. *Fertil. Steril.* 47:1025, 1987.
32. Matson, P. L., and Yovich, J. L. Gamete intrafallopian transfer in a non-IVF unit. *Lancet* 1:112, 1987.
33. Matson, P. L., et al. The in vitro fertilization of supernumerary oocytes in a gamete intrafallopian transfer program. *Fertil. Steril.* 47:802, 1987.
34. Matson, P. L., et al. The role of gamete intrafallopian transfer (GIFT) in the treatment of oligospermic infertility. *Fertil. Steril.* 48:608, 1987.
35. McGaughey, R. W., and Nemiro, J. S. Correlation of estrogen levels with oocytes aspirated and with pregnancy in a program of clinical tubal transfer. *Fertil. Steril.* 48:98, 1987.
36. Medical Research International, American Fertility Society Special Interest Group. In vitro fertilization/embryo transfer in the United States: 1985 and 1986 results from the national IVF-ET Registry. *Fertil. Steril.* 49:212, 1988.
37. Molloy, D., et al. Laparoscopic approach to a program of gamete intrafallopian transfer. *Fertil. Steril.* 47:289, 1987.
38. Nemiro, J. S., and McGaughey, R. W. An alternative to in vitro fertilization-embryo transfer: The success of human oocytes and spermatozoa to the distal oviduct. *Fertil. Steril.* 46:644, 1986.
39. Olive, D. L., et al. Gamete intrafallopian intrauterine transfer (GIFT) complicated by bilateral ectopic pregnancy. *Fertil. Steril.* 49:719, 1988.
40. Pavlou, C., and Pampiglione, J. Gamete intrafallopian transfer in a non-IVF unit. *Lancet* 2:1152, 1986.
41. Quigley, M. M., et al. Simultaneous in vitro fertilization and gamete intrafallopian transfer (GIFT). *Fertil. Steril.* 47:797, 1987.
42. Serhal, P. F., et al. Unexplained infertility—the value of Pergonal superovulation combined with intrauterine insemination. *Fertil. Steril.* 49:602, 1988.
43. Shettles, L. B. Ova harvest with in vivo fertilization. *Am. J. Obstet. Gynecol.* 133:845, 1979.
44. Steptoe, P. C., and Edwards, R. G. Birth after the reimplantation of a human embryo. *Lancet* 2:366, 1978.
45. Tesarik, J., et al. Oocyte recovery, in vitro insemination, and transfer into the oviduct after its microsurgical repair at a single laparotomy. *Fertil. Steril.* 39:472, 1983.
46. Van der Ven, H. H., et al. Polyspermia in in vitro fertilization of human oocytes: Frequency and possible causes. *Ann. N.Y. Acad. Sci.* 442:88, 1985.
47. Wurfel, W., et al. Pregnancy after intratubal gamete transfer via hysteroscopy. *Geburtshilfe Frauenheilkd* 48:401, 1988.
48. Yovich, J. L., and Matson, P. L. Pregnancy rates after high intrauterine insemination of husband's spermatozoa or gamete intrafallopian transfer. *Lancet* 2:1287, 1986.
49. Yovich, J. L., et al. Pregnancies following pronuclear stage tubal transfer. *Fertil. Steril.* 48:851, 1987.

50. Yovich, J. L., et al. The treatment of normospermic infertility by gamete intra-fallopian transfer (GIFT). *Br. J. Obstet. Gynaecol.* 95:361, 1988.
51. Yovich, J. L., Yovich, J. M., and Eidrisinghe, W. R. The relative chance of pregnancy following tubal or uterine transfer procedures. *Fertil. Steril.* 49:858, 1988.

# Cryopreservation in a Human IVF Program

## Lynette Wilson

With the increased success rates of ovarian stimulation, oocyte retrieval, and in vitro fertilization and development, the problem of dealing with excess oocytes and embryos has arisen. Again, as the whole field of assisted reproduction expands, the number of cases presenting for oocyte donation is also increasing. In both instances a need for oocyte and embryo freezing arises. In the first instance, excess embryos from one induction cycle could be held in storage for later use by the couple, should the initial embryo transfer be unsuccessful, or for later attempts at a second or third pregnancy. Freezing deals both with the problem of excess embryos and offers a simple way for a couple to have multiple embryo transfers from only one stimulation cycle. In the case of oocyte donation, a bank of oocytes could be established in much the same way as sperm banks have been. Thus, women requiring oocyte donation could be better matched with a donor oocyte, and the procedures of timing for embryo replacement could be tailored to the recipient rather than being governed by the donor. Alternatively, the donor oocytes could be fertilized with the recipient husband's sperm, grown in vitro, and then frozen as cleaving embryos. Again, the embryo replacement could be better timed and controlled.

Though cryopreservation is not a new technique, only in the past 15 years has the field developed to a point where these issues can actually be contemplated. The development of freezing techniques to successfully cryopreserve mammalian tissue in a viable form began in the 1940s. In 1949 Polge, Smith, and Parkes[7] reported the first attempts at successfully cryopreserving avian spermatozoa. The cryoprotectant they used was glycerol. From this point the science of sperm freezing developed, with successful techniques and sperm banks being developed for many species. Techniques for cryopreservation of the female gametes or the developing zygote followed slowly with an initial unsuccessful attempt in 1953 by Smith (17). Glycerol was used to cryopreserve mouse embryos, but only 1% survived. It was not until 1972 that the techniques to freeze, thaw, grow, and implant mouse embryos were established (21,23,24). Since then the number of species for which it is possible to successfully freeze and thaw preimplantation embryos has increased to include humans, with the first success being reported in 1983 (18). The techniques have also developed and altered as the actual dynamics of oocyte and embryo freezing have been elucidated. Though much of the initial freezing experiments on embryos and oocytes were conducted on the mouse model, the general principles have been adapted to allow the zygotes of other species to be frozen successfully; however, much of the data collected on any one species have been empiric, and this is very important when the differences in size, in vitro culture characteristics, zona thickness, temperature sensitivity, and temperature coefficient are compared in oocytes and embryos. Combined, these characteristics influence both the methods of freezing and thawing and how the embryo will respond and survive.

## PRINCIPLES OF CRYOPRESERVATION

Whether one is dealing with a single cell, as in unfertilized oocytes and pronuclear stage fertilized embryos, or with a multiblastomer cleaving embryo, the same principles apply for the effects of cryoprotectant and decreasing temperature. For this reason the following discussion deals with a single spherical cell, be it oocyte or individual blastomer.

Cells comprise a large pool of water and, when being handled in vitro, are suspended in an aqueous medium. As water is cooled it will begin to freeze, and it has been shown that the physical damage caused by ice in both the freezing and thawing procedures is what is most likely to damage the cells (8,11,12). To overcome this, a *cryoprotectant* is used. A cryoprotectant is described as a substance that can replace water in the cell and afford protection from ice damage. Exactly how the cryoprotectants work is still not precisely known, but it has been suggested that they act in a colligative manner to reduce electrolyte concentrations within each cell at subzero temperatures (16). Many cryoprotectants have been successfully used in different freezing protocols: alone, in combination with sucrose, or in so-called cocktails of cryoprotectants.

When an oocyte or embryo is placed into the cryoprotectant, it will begin to shrink because it will lose water to the external hyperosmotic solution. This is aided by the cell membrane, which is more permeable to water than cryoprotectant. Slowly cryoprotectant will enter the cells and an equilibrium will be reached when the loss of water and influx of cryoprotectant are equal. At this point shrinkage stops. The cryoprotectant will enter the cell at a rate dependent on its permeability. This is described as how fast it can pass through a membrane (permeability coefficient), the temperature coefficient, and the concentration. As the working temperature increases, the temperature coefficient increases and hence the permeability. It therefore takes glycerol 10 times longer to reach equilibrium with mouse eight-cell embryos at 0°C than at 22°C (16). The greater the permeability the better; however, warming to afford increases is inadvisable as certain cryopreservatives have been shown to be toxic at higher temperatures. The permeability of any one cryoprotectant will alter with cell type (species), cell stage, cell size, and temperature and is generally empirically derived for any individual system. Once the cells are equilibrated with cryoprotectant, the freezing phases can begin, and these can be accomplished in one of three ways (20,21,22,23,24): slow (8,22), fast (20,22), and rapid (19,25), including vitrification (9,10,13).

## Slow and Fast Freezing

With slow and fast freezing, five phases can be identified. In the *prefreeze stage* the cells that are fully equilibrated with the chosen cryoprotectant are cooled to a temperature of approximately $-6- -10°C$ for induction of ice nucleation or seeding. It is necessary to stimulate ice formation with these solutions as they tend to supercool to low subzero temperatures where they spontaneously form ice, and the cells are damaged. Ice induction can be accomplished by either touching the freezing vessel with chilled forceps, introducing an ice crystal as a nucleus, or by vibrations caused by gently tapping the freezing vessel. With *seeding,* the first phase transition occurs. As ice forms around the cell, the latent heat of fusion is released, which raises the temperature of the solution, hence the need to "hold" the freezing system at the seeding temperature for a period, to allow it to recool to the seeding temperature.

As ice forms within the external solution, the concentration of solutes in the now partially frozen solute will increase. More ice will form until the chemical potential of the water in the unfrozen fraction reaches an equilibrium with the chemical potential of ice. As this is a direct function of the temperature, more ice will form the lower the temperature gets until the whole sample is frozen. As the concentration of solutes in the external unfrozen solute increases, the cells will lose more of their unfrozen water down the concentration gradient and hence shrink further. The hold at the seeding temperature allows this process to be completed. At equilibrium the intracellular chemical potential is equivalent to that in the unfrozen extracellular substrate. The relatively large volume of intracellular water in oocytes and preimplantation embryos, when compared with other cells, is the major factor in the need to seed.

After seeding and a hold for re-equilibration, the *freezing phase* can begin. This is accomplished by slowly (0.13°C/minute) lowering the temperature. This very slow rate of cooling is required because of the physical properties of embryos and oocytes. First, water has a low permeability in embryos, and this is emphasized by the low surface area–volume ratio. As the unfrozen water in the external medium continues to freeze, a chemical potential between it and the supercooled water in the cells is established so more water leaves the cells and freezes externally. By keeping the cooling rates slow, this process is accomplished gradually, thereby avoiding cellular damage or intracellular ice formation. Higher cooling rates will result in more heat than water transport, leaving too much intracellular water to form ice, which will damage the cell. In a slow-cool program, this cooling is continued to $-80°C$ before rapid transfer to liquid nitrogen. At this point the cells have dehydrated to the maximum and have no intracellular ice. A fast-cool program terminates the cooling phase at approximately $-30--40°C$ before plunging into liquid nitrogen. As full dehydration has not occurred, either small ice crystals will form within the cell, or a glassy unstable state is established. In both instances embryos may be *stored* in their frozen state indefinitely with little possibility of genetic damage or alteration from background radiation.

After storage, the *thawing phase* occurs. The method of freezing, i.e., slow or fast, governs the thawing procedures (20). Embryos, cells, and oocytes frozen by the slow method require slow thawing, at a rate of approximately $8°C$/minute to room temperature at which point the cryoprotectant is diluted out. During this slow thaw, the cells can gradually rehydrate without ice formation, in a reverse process to that experienced with freezing. If the thaw is too rapid, they will experience massive osmotic shock, which will irreparably damage them. Cells frozen by the fast method require a very rapid thawing procedure. The freezing vials are removed from liquid nitrogen ($-196°C$) and placed immediately in a $37°C$ water bath. This effects an almost instant thawing, which prevents any intracellular ice that has formed during freezing from damaging the cell. As these embryos were only partially dehydrated, unlike those in the slow-cool method, they will not suffer the large and damaging osmotic shock caused by very rapid dehydration. Again the cryoprotectant can be diluted out, leaving the embryos ready for in vitro culture or implantation, or both.

### Rapid Freezing or Vitrification

Rapid freezing and vitrification have only two major phases: freezing and thawing. In vitrification a mixture of cryoprotectants is used (3,9,10), whereas high concentrations of dimethyl sulphoxide (DMSO) and sucrose are used for rapid freezing (19,25). As the concentrations of cryoprotectants are very high, cells shrink extremely fast due to a very rapid loss of water to the external hyperosmotic system. Within minutes of placing the cells into the cryoprotectant, they are plunged directly into liquid nitrogen. It is thought that in both instances, a glassy intracellular state is formed (19). Thawing in both instances is rapid, accomplished by placing the freezing vessel into a water bath at $37°C$ immediately on removal from liquid nitrogen. Embryos and oocytes frozen in this manner are viable in vitro, but large fetal losses after transfer have been reported (13). To avoid this, in the mouse system, with good implantation and fetal growth rates, a very slow removal of the cryoprotectants is required (25).

## CRYOPROTECTANTS, MEDIA, FREEZING MACHINES, AND VESSELS IN CRYOPRESERVATION

Many substances have been used for the cryopreservation of mammalian oocytes and embryos, most commonly DMSO, propanediol, and glycerol. Currently propanediol is the favored cryoprotectant for the fast methods of embryo freezing (6,14) as it has been shown to be less toxic than DMSO (14) and allows intracellular ice formation; however, DMSO has been more successfully employed in the freezing of oocytes in both humans (1) and mice (26). For the slow methods using either embryos or oocytes, DMSO has to be used. Although glycerol was one of the first cryoprotectants to be used, its use is now limited to the freezing of blastocysts (2,4). As it has a very low permeability coefficient, it cannot effectively replace water in large cells that have a low surface area–volume ratio, but the cells in blastocysts are small enough to have high surface area–volume ratios and can therefore fully equilibrate with glycerol at room temperature. Glycerol has also been shown to be the best cryoprotectant for the freezing of blastocysts. The use of sucrose in freezing or thawing solutions, or both, helps protect the cells from swelling by acting as an osmotic balance. It is more important in thawing, where it prevents too rapid a rehydration. During the freezing phase, it slows the dehydration, allowing gradual shrinkage, again protecting the cells from damaging rapid fluxes (5).

Various culture media have been employed in freezing protocols and tend to be chosen by availability and ease of access; however, the use of a phosphate buffered medium is not recommended as it has been shown that although embryos survive the freeze-thaw process, they are unable to resume development. It is not understood what causes this phenomenon. Bicarbonate buffered media are also not recommended because of the difficulty in controlling the pH. On the bench they will become very alkaline and then gradually more acidic as the temperature drops and more carbon dioxide is dissolved. It is therefore best to employ a Hepes buffered medium (20–25 mM). All freezing solutions should contain protein, either as heat-inactivated serum (15%) or bovine serum albumin (5 mg/ml Sigma Fract V No. A9647).

The choice of freezing vessel is usually governed by the machine being employed and the freezing protocol being used. Various sizes of both glass vials and plastic straws have been successfully used. Small plastic straws are recommended because they offer an environment with a small volume of external medium, which reduces the stress and shearing forces on the embryos caused by the ice crystals (15). They are also easier to store in large numbers.

Currently many freezing machines are on the market, using many different principles to effect a cooling curve. The three most popular, using a liquid nitrogen gas phase, are the Cryomed, Planar, and Minicool. All are adequate, have reproducible cooling curves, and are widely used. The Planar and Minicool have automatic seeding devices, which need to be monitored very carefully as seeding does not always occur (26). The Cryomed employs manual seeding. One major drawback with all three machines is that they operate on a gas phase, which means that the removal or introduction of straws/vials, seeding, and so forth can cause large gas displacements and currents and therefore large temperature fluctuations. Machines that operate on baths of cooled liquid, such as 100% ethanol, afford a much more stable cooling environment. An excellent machine in this group is the Biocool. In all machines an automatic device lowers the temperature at the programmed rate, with holds and seeding phases. Control vials/straws containing a thermocouple and linked to a recorder give visual indication of what the temperature curve looks like in the freezing vessels.

Storage, after freezing, should be in a liquid nitrogen container specifically set aside for this purpose. It is highly detrimental to frozen oocytes and embryos to experience any temperature fluctuations before thawing. Straws and vials should never be lifted out of the liquid nitrogen until the point of thawing.

## REFERENCES

1. Chen, C. Pregnancy after human oocyte cryopreservation. *Lancet* 19:884, 1986.
2. Cohen, J., et al. Pregnancies following the frozen storage of expanding human blastocysts. *J. In Vitro Fert. Embryo Transf.* 2:59, 1985.
3. Fahy, G. M., et al. Vitrification as an approach to cryopreservation. *Cryobiology* 21:407, 1984.
4. Fehilly, C. B., et al. Cryopreservation of cleaving embryos and expanded blastocyst in the human: a comparative study. *Fertil. Steril.* 44:638, 1985.
5. Kasai, M., Niwa, K., and Iritani, A. Protective effect of sucrose on the survival of mouse and rat embryos stored at 0°C. *J. Reprod. Fertil.* 68:377, 1983.

6. Lassale, B., Testart, J., and Renard, J. P. Human embryo features that influence the success of cryopreservation with the use of 1-2 propanediol. *Fertil. Steril.* 44:645, 1985.

7. Polge, C., Smith A. U., and Parkes, A. S. Revival of spermatozoa after vitrification and dehydration at low temperature. *Nature* 164:666, 1949.

8. Rall, W. F. The role of intracellular ice in the slow warming injury of mouse embryos. In G. H. Zielmaker (Ed.). *Frozen Storage of Laboratory Animals* New York: Gustav Fischer Verlag, 1981. Pp. 33–34.

9. Rall, W. F., and Fahy, G. M. Ice-free cryopreservation of mouse embryos at − 196°C by vitrification. *Nature* 313:573, 1985.

10. Rall, W. F., and Fahy, G. M. Vitrification: A new approach to embryo cryopreservation. *Theriogenology* 13:1, 220, 1985.

11. Rall, W. T., Reid, D. S., and Farrant, J. Innocuous biological freezing during warming. *Nature* 286:511, 1980.

12. Rall, W. F., Reid, D. S., and Polge, C. Analysis of slow warming injury of mouse embryos by cryomicroscopical and physiochemical methods. *Cryobiology* 21:106, 1984.

13. Rall, W. F., et al. Development of mouse embryos cryopreserved by vitrification. *J. Reprod. Fertil.* 80:499, 1987.

14. Renard, J. P. The cryopreservation of mammalian embryos. Human in vitro fertilization. *INSERM* Symposium, No. 24:201–208, 1985.

15. Renard, J. P., and Babinet, C. High survival of mouse embryos after rapid freezing and thawing inside plastic straws with 1-2 propanediol as cryoprotectant. *J. Exp. Zool.* 230:443, 1984.

16. Schneider, U. Cryobiological principles of embryo freezing. *J. In Vitro Fert. Embryo Transf.* 3:3, 1986.

17. Smith, A. U. Discussion on the survival of tissues at low temperatures. *Proceedings of the Royal Society of Medicine.* 47:57–60, 1953.

18. Trounson, A., and Mohr, L. Human pregnancy following cryopreservation, thawing and transfer of an eight-cell embryo. *Nature* 305:707, 1983.

19. Trounson, A., Peura, A., and Kirby, C. Ultrarapid freezing: A new low cost and effective method of embryo cryopreservation. *Fertil. Steril.* 48:843, 1987.

20. Whittingham, D. G. Principles of embryo preservation. In M. J. Ashwood-Smith and J. Farrant (eds.), *Low Temperature Preservation in Medicine and Biology.* Chap. 4, pp. 65–83.

21. Whittingham, D. G. The survival of mouse embryos after freezing and thawing. *Nature* 233:125–126, 1971.

22. Whittingham, D. G., et al. Survival of frozen mouse embryos after rapid thawing from − 196°C. *J. Reprod. Fertil.* 56:11, 1979.

23. Whittingham, D. G., Leibo, S. P., and Mazur, P. Survival of mouse embryos frozen to − 196°C and − 269°C. *Science* 178:411, 1972.

24. Wilmut, I. The effect of cooling rate, warming rate, cryoprotective agent and stage of development on survival of mouse embryos during freezing and thawing. *Life Sci.* 11:1071, 1972.

25. Wilson, L. A., and Quinn, P. Development of mouse embryos cryopreserved by an ultra rapid method of freezing. *Hum. Reprod.* 4(1):86–90, 1989.

26. Wilson, L. A., et al. Cryopreservation of mouse oocytes and pronuclear stage embryos: The effects of post-ovulatory age, cryoprotectant and freezing methodology. *J. In Vitro Fert. Embryo Transf.* (In press).

# Appendix 13-1.  Protocol for Human Blastocyst Freezing

**FREEZING SOLUTIONS**
Solution 1:   20% human serum (HS) in medium (M),
              i.e., 16 ml M + 4 ml HS
Solution 2:   16% glycerol (G) in M + 20% HS,
              i.e., 0.8 ml G + 4.2 ml sol. 1

Make the following solutions and place in 35-mm culture dishes:

|   | %9 | ml Sol. 2 | ml Sol. 1 |
|---|----|-----------|-----------|
| a | 1  | 0.2       | 2.8       |
| b | 2  | 0.4       | 2.6       |
| c | 4  | 0.8       | 2.2       |
| d | 6  | 1.1       | 1.9       |
| e | 8  | 1.5       | 1.5       |

Blastocysts are placed for 10 min in each concentration of G. They are then loaded into the freezing vessel containing 8% G in M + 20% HS (sol. e) placed in the freezing machine, which is cooled at a rate of 1°C/min to $-6-\!-10°C$. Hold at this temperature for 5 min during which time seeding is accomplished. The cooling phase can then begin with a cooling rate of 0.33°C/min to $-30°C$. At this temperature the freezing vessels are placed directly into liquid nitrogen with as little exposure to temperature changes as possible.

**THAWING SOLUTION**
16% G in M with 20% HS, i.e., sol. 2
Require 8, 6, 5, 4, 3, 2, 1% glycerol solutions

i.e., sol. e, d, c, b, a, f, g

| plus | ml Sol. 2 | ml Sol. 2 |
|------|-----------|-----------|
| 5%   | − f − 0.9 | 2.1       |
| 3%   | − g − 0.6 | 2.4       |

All solutions are placed in 35-mm dishes. Freezing vessels are removed from the liquid nitrogen, agitated rapidly in a water bath at $+37°C$, and, just as the last ice crystals disappear, removed to room temperature.

The blastocysts are then expelled into 8% G, i.e., sol. e for 10 min, sol. d for 12 min, sol. f for 14 min, sol. c for 16 min, sol. g for 18 min, sol. b for 20 min, and finally sol. a for 20 min. They are then washed 3 times in M + 20% HS and slowly warmed to 37°C. At this point they will begin to expand if they have collapsed. They can then be used in embryo transfer.

For more effective thawing, the addition of 0.2 M sucrose to all the thawing solutions is recommended. This can be removed in the final washing steps.

From G. M. Fahy et al. Vitrification as an approach to cryoperservation. *Cryobiology* 21:407, 1984; C. B. Fehilly et al. Cryopreservation of cleaving embryos and expanded blastocyst in the human: a comparative study. *Fertil. Steril.* 44:638, 1985.

# Appendix 13-2.  Pronuclear Stage and Cleaving Embryo Freezing: Propanediol and Sucrose Method

## FREEZING SOLUTIONS

(1)   20 ml medium (M) + 20% human serum (HS), i.e., 16 ml M + 4 ml HS
(2)   1.5 M propanediol (PD) in M + 20% HS, i.e., 10 ml sol. 1 + 1.25 ml PD
(3)   1.5 M PD + 20% HS + 0.2 M sucrose, i.e., 5 ml sol. 2 + 0.342 gm sucrose

Prepare the following and place in small 35-mm culture dishes:

|            | ml Sol. 2 | ml Sol. 1 |
|------------|-----------|-----------|
| 0.5 MPD — a | 1 | 2 |
| 1.0 MPD — b | 2 | 1 |
| 1.5 MPD — c | 3 | 0 |

At room temperature, place the embryos in sol. a for 5 min, followed by sol. b for 5 min, followed by sol. c for 10 min. Then transfer them into the freezing container containing sol. 3, place them in the freezing machine, and begin cooling at a rate of 2°C/min from room temperature to $-6-10$°C. Hold at this temperature for 10 min during which time seeding is accomplished (after approximately 3–5 min). Then begin the cooling phase by lowering the temperature at 0.33°C/min until $-30$°C. At this point the freezing vials are placed directly into liquid nitrogen, with as little temperature fluctuation as possible. Freezing vessels should contain ideally one embryo, but never more than two. They can be attached to metal canes for storage in the liquid nitrogen tank.

## THAWING SOLUTIONS

(1)   15 ml M + 20% HS, i.e., 12 ml M + 3 ml HS
(2)   M + 0.2 M sucrose, i.e., 8 ml M + 0.548 gm sucrose
(3)   M + 0.2 M sucrose + 1.5 MPD, i.e., 5 ml sol. 1 + 0.63 ml PD + 0.385 gm sucrose

Prepare the following and place in small 35-mm culture dishes:

| MPD |   | ml Sol. 3 | ml Sol. 2 |
|-----|---|-----------|-----------|
| 1.0 | a | 2 | 1 |
| 0.5 | b | 1 | 2 |

Straws are removed from the liquid nitrogen, agitated rapidly in a water bath at $+37$°C, and, just as the last ice vanishes, removed to room temperature. The embryos are then expelled from the vessel into a dish containing sol. a. After 5 min they are moved to sol. b, left for 5 min, and then moved into sol. a2, i.e., 0.2 M sucrose in M with 20% HS. After 5–10 min in this solution, they are washed 3 times in M = 20% HS, i.e., sol. 1, and either used in embryo transfer or placed in culture in the incubator.

B. Lassale, J. Testart, and J. P. Renard. Human embryo features that influence the success of cryopreservation with the use of 1-2 propanediol. *Fertil. Steril.* 44:645, 1985.

# Current Considerations in Assisted Reproductive Technologies

# Ethical Aspects of IVF and Related Assisted Reproductive Technologies

## Edward E. Wallach

The frequency of infertility in the United States has been estimated at 15% of the population in the reproductive age range. Based on a population in this age group in the United States, approximately 10 million Americans have a problem establishing a pregnancy in any point in time. Of this figure approximately 15% of couples never even have an obvious cause uncovered to explain their infertility. Many or both of these groups consider the possibility of or become candidates for in vitro fertilization (IVF) or another of the modern-day means used to assist conception.

Current-day modalities that deviate from conventional approaches to reproduction include

1. Artificial placement of sperm (see various techniques discussed in this chapter)
2. Artificial placement of sperm and egg
3. Extracorporeal fertilization and pre-embryo replacement (IVF)
4. Gamete donation
   a. Sperm
   b. Ovum
5. Embryo donation
6. Surrogacy
   a. Gestational mother
   b. Ovum donor/gestational mother
7. Cryopreservation
   a. Gamete
   b. Embryo
8. Micromanipulation of ovum or embryo

For many years observations conducted on animals have formed a basis for treating human infertility with these modalities. Such extensively used procedures as artificial insemination (AI) and IVF were not only first successfully accomplished in animals, but have subsequently become more or less state-of-the-art procedures in animal husbandry. These procedures, when applied to the cattle industry, are viewed from two vantage points: nutrition and economics. Reproductive interventions among farm animals are of critical value to human well-being not only for these two reasons, but also for the techniques themselves, which may be extrapolated to their use in humans; however, for "ethical" or "moral" reasons, procedures involving manipulation of normal reproductive processes are not as widely accepted in humans as they are in the laboratory or farm animals. Freed from the ethical limitations surrounding the "new" reproductive technologies in humans and based on bottom-line economics, professionals in the field of animal husbandry have established the groundwork for techniques now being applied for correction of infertility in humans. The actual implementation of AI in breeding of livestock, in fact, preceded its use in humans by 4 centuries. It was not until 1884 that William Pancoast from Philadelphia described the first donor insemination on record in the United States. In humans we must maintain a degree of societal equilibrium not required in animals, as well as a high level of respect for limits on what is morally and ethically acceptable. To be able to alleviate infertility without ignoring the human element in the conception and childbearing processes and without offending society is a high priority principle.

The birth of baby Louise Brown in 1978 escalated public awareness of the ethical issues surrounding third-party involvement in the reproductive process and in the application of assisted reproductive technology. The medical community rapidly grasped this opportunity to transform IVF from the realm of experimentation to that of clinical practice. The modifying terms of *research* and *experimental* connote the unknown and its attendant risks, whereas the realities of IVF permit the incorporation of a clinically applicable procedure into general usage, a concept that has great appeal to the competitive and entrepreneurial spirit of many individuals in our society. Because of rapid advances in reproductive methodology, the feeling has prevailed that science and technology have gotten uncomfortably ahead of our ability to interpret, individualize, and regulate IVF and related procedures.

## ETHICS OF NEW REPRODUCTIVE TECHNOLOGIES

This section is designed to provide the practicing physician with a framework for viewing "new reproductive technologies," many of which are not actually so "new" within the perspective of acceptability. What defines the ethical substance of an action? The often-used term *ethics* defies a universally acceptable definition. Contained within the framework of reaching an ethical decision are many variables: utility, religious influences, actions that seem natural or appropriate, the pressures or commitments to one's own vocation or profession, legal limitations, and peer pressure, among others. Ultimately each of these considerations and many others impact on one's judgment as to whether an action is ethically right or wrong. Compounding these considerations in the United States is the very nature of our culture, which has been pointedly pluralistic since its establishment over 2 centuries ago. "The human person integrally and adequately considered" implies the sum of all dimensions of a given individual that lead him or her to render an ethical judgment (1). Three ethical principles represent the underpinnings of moral judgments:

1. *The concepts of beneficence and nonmaleficence* or doing no harm while promoting societal welfare—the utilitarian approach
2. *Respect for autonomy,* in which the individual has the right to control his or her own destiny—the libertarian credo
3. *Justice* as an arbiter between liberties and distribution of risk-benefit ratios. How these liberties are awarded to individuals raises additional ethical problems. Are they awarded to everyone according to merit, to everyone according to need, to everyone equally, or to everyone according to what has been acquired by proper means?—the egalitarian principle

Furthermore, of necessity, a stratification exists in the levels at which regulation, guidelines, or ethical types of decisions can be developed and implemented in our society. They can be developed by the patient or consumer; they can be developed by the physician, scientist, or provider, or combinations thereof; they can also be developed by ethics committees or review boards that ideally consist of representatives whose functions would be to balance the needs of the patient on one hand, and the modalities provided by physician/scientist on the other, blended with those standards held by the society in which they function. Once guidelines and standards have been established, implementation or adherence is further enforced either by legislation or by threat of litigation for infractions of the law or for inflicting harm. These regulatory strata function reasonably well to maintain order for nonmedical services or even medical services that do not encompass reproductive technology. Combinations of laws governing safety, licensing requirements, professional or trade associations, consumer pressures, and institutional review boards interact effectively to protect the user/consumer of all varieties of services. Reproductive technology, however, falls into a unique category for at least two reasons: (1) sexuality and procreation have a special meaning among all persons and are reinfluenced by beliefs of different religious groups; (2) the field of assisted reproductive technology has advanced so rapidly over the past decade that in many instances procedures that should have been preceded by clearly defined risks and benefits to society as well as to the individual have been rapidly implemented. As a result, these procedures run the risk of offending society and evoking a reaction that may impose stringent restrictions on their use. In contrast guidelines can be so rigid that they stifle creativity and halt progress in areas in which scientific help is needed.

Based on the source of gametes (homologous or donor for both members of the couple), the site of fertilization (wife, laboratory, surrogate), the carrier of the pregnancy (wife, surrogate), 16 alternatives can be identified resulting in the human (Table 14-1). By factoring in cryopreservation of gametes or embryos, these possibilities can be extended even further. To invoke any of these procedures as adjuncts in infertility treatment either individually or in combination, and to provide clear access to their use, society must determine whether an individual has a legal right to reproduce. In the United States, the Supreme Court has viewed reproductive liberty in two contexts: the illegality of imposing sterilization on a criminal, and the freedom of an individual's access to contraceptive measures. When viewed from the vantage point of curtailment of reproductive function, these governmental affirmations of the individual's freedom to his or her reproductive rights clearly define the principle of procreative liberty. To interpret this concept further, one needs to question whether the right to procreative liberty applies to the unmarried individual as well as to the married person or couple and whether it pertains to noncoital methods for reproduction as well as to conventional means of reproduction. For example, if an unmarried woman is entitled to use contraception for pregnancy prevention, should she also be entitled to a right to conceive? Whenever noncoital methodology needs to be applied, involvement of a third party, separation of the coital act from conception, and removal of the conjugal from the procreative aspects of reproduction enter the equation. These latter considerations represent the basis for Catholicism's objection to use of the new reproductive technologies.

Throughout the world, techniques in assisted reproduction have been evaluated, such as the Warnock Committee Report in Great Britain (5); the Victoria Committee to Consider the Social, Ethical and Legal Issues Arising from In Vitro Fertilization (the Waller Committee Report), in Australia (6); the Ontario Law Reform Commission's Report on Human Artificial Reproduction and Related Matters, in Canada (3); and the American Fertility Society's Ethics Committee Report entitled "Ethical Considerations of the New Reproductive Technologies" (1).

## IN VITRO FERTILIZATION

IVF was originally devised as a means to bypass fallopian tubes that are damaged or absent, by substituting the laboratory as a site for fertilization. Obtaining and transporting gametes to a culture system that can support fertilization and then conveying the product of fertilization to the mother's uterus do away with the necessity for the fallopian tube in the conception process. The indications for IVF have ultimately broadened, by virtue of the success of the basic procedure, to encompass oligospermia, endometriosis, and long-standing infertility without any identifiable cause. Although the technique has become an integral part of various modalities now widely available for infertile couples, a number of reservations still exist regarding the IVF procedure. Since it separates procreations from sexual union, IVF has not been deemed acceptable by the Roman Catholic Church. Despite the birth of thousands of offspring around the world through IVF, concern still persists regarding the possible impairment in quality of offspring through gamete manipulation. Given the simplicity of the principle, fear that this technique will be abused or lead to less acceptable reproductive technologies provides the basis for the slippery-slope concept. This concept implies that one innovation of necessity leads to another, the latter

Table 14-1. Alternate methods of reproduction

| Gamete male | Source female | Fertilization site | Pregnancy site | Comments |
|---|---|---|---|---|
| H | W | W | W | Natural, AIH, GIFT |
| S | W | W | W | AID |
| H | W | L | W | IVF, ZIFT, PROST |
| S | W | L | W | IVF, ZIFT, PROST, donor sperm |
| H | S | L | W | IVF, ZIFT, PROST, donor egg |
| S | S | L | W | IVF, ZIFT, PROST, donor gametes, or donor embryo |
| H | S | S | W | AIH/donor woman plus uterine lavage |
| S | S | S | W | AID/donor woman plus uterine lavage |
| H | W | W | S | Surrogate motherhood |
| S | W | L | S | Surrogate motherhood |
| H | W | L | S | Surrogate motherhood |
| S | W | L | S | Surrogate motherhood |
| H | S | L | S | Surrogate motherhood |
| S | S | S | S | Surrogate motherhood |
| H | S | S | S | Surrogate motherhood |
| S | S | S | S | Surrogate motherhood |

H, husband; W, wife; S, third party (substitute or surrogate); L, laboratory; ZIFT, zygote intrafallopian transfer; PROST, pronuclear stage ovum transfer; GIFT, gamete intrafallopian transfer.

**Table 14-2. Indications for AID**

Azoospermia
Irreversible sterilization by vasectomy
Uncorrectable abnormalities in semen
Genetic disorders
Ejaculatory dysfunction
Mutagenic exposure

being less palatable than the former. Furthermore, one of the issues that has not yet been completely addressed involves concern that the procedure is both elective and costly. IVF is, therefore, not available to everyone equally. Furthermore, the concern has been voiced that through IVF, limited resources are being used inappropriately at great expense to provide more offspring to an already overpopulated world. Concerns over contributing to unbridled population growth, however, rarely, if ever deter any given infertile couple in its quest for a child.

## HOMOLOGOUS TECHNIQUES

### Artificial Insemination

Artificial insemination with husband semen (AIH) has been used for many years, primarily in situations in which natural insemination is not possible or is deemed inefficient. Obviously, AIH is an integral component of IVF since the manner in which fertilization occurs necessitates artificial placement of spermatozoa; however, because techniques entail the preparation and calibration of sperm prior to their addition to the oocyte in the laboratory, sperm washing techniques for AIH have become standardized and used routinely whenever intrauterine insemination (IUI) is performed. With ease and standardization of techniques such as AIH, the hazard always exists that indications will become extended beyond what is logical and the procedure will be abused. For example, is a diagnosis of "unexplained infertility" grounds for using AIH when normal insemination has been documented through postcoital testing? With techniques already developed claiming successful separation of X- and Y-bearing sperm, is sex selection a justifiable adjunct to assisted reproductive technology? If sperm separation techniques are ethically acceptable, under what circumstances should they be used? Should use of this technology be restricted to attempts at avoiding sex-linked genetic disorders, or should sex selection techniques be available to all families on request? It is unrealistic to expect that a procedure such as manipulation of semen to achieve sex selection can ever be regulated. Like IVF, the technology involved in AIH separates procreation from sexual expression and, as such, is not acceptable to the Catholic Church.

### Artificial Donor Insemination

Artificial insemination using the semen of a third party (AID) has been a widely acceptable procedure since its initial use in humans about a century ago. Indications for its use are listed in Table 14-2.

The donor insemination procedure maintains both genetic and gestational links to the mother. AID has become widely used currently. The relative scarcity of adoptable infants has heightened the demand for AID among couples with male factor infertility. Furthermore, most stigmas originally associated with AID have faded in the light of positive publicity and widespread use. The use of donor sperm in the IVF process parallels indications for AID in general. In contrast to AIH and to conventional IVF, AID introduces a new variable, namely the incorporation of a third party into the reproductive process. Increasing concerns about dissemination of sexually transmitted diseases have prompted principles to minimize the possibility that donor sperm will serve as the vector. These

**Table 14-3. Potential sources of donor oocytes**

Incidental at time of surgery
Excess oocytes during IVF procedures
Relative
Friend

include careful screening of donors and quarantine of semen samples through cryopreservation during which time prolonged testing of aliquots can be accomplished. Although evaluation of the donor semen for sexually transmitted diseases can be performed with ease, screening to completely exclude genetic disorders is more difficult to accomplish. Anonymity of the donor is customarily maintained, but if an inherited abnormality in the offspring should be uncovered after birth, the physician is committed to pursue the donor and inform him of the adverse genetic outcome in an attempt to protect his personal reproductive future. AID has been used long enough to have enabled states to adopt laws regarding responsibility for the paternity of all offspring resulting from AID. In general, the spouse of the inseminated woman is considered the legal father. Questions regarding psychological effects on the product of asymmetric parenthood have never been resolved, but to date there is no indication of adverse effects of AID on the offspring. Finally, donor sperm can also be considered as a backup measure in IVF, if the husband were to be unable to provide a specimen after oocyte retrieval or should the oocytes obtained fail to be fertilized by the husband's sperm. The couple undergoing IVF must be carefully prepared and counselled before resorting to the use of donor sperm in these cases. Use of donor sperm in an IVF program carries with it reservations similar to those for AID or IVF when performed as independent procedures. Caution must be applied when considering "backup" sperm for use in an IVF program following apparent failed fertilization by the husband's sperm with respect to paternity of offspring and to the possible consequences of fertilization delay and aging of oocytes.

**Oocyte Donation**

The need for donor oocytes might arise in patients who lack ovaries (e.g., ovarian agenesis or previous surgical extirpation) and in patients with ovarian failure. Parallel to the indications for donor sperm, donor oocytes can be used to avoid transmission of known genetic defects from mother to offspring. Occasionally oocyte retrieval may be so technically difficult that use of donor oocytes is necessitated. Because oocyte donation requires delicate coordination between cycle of the donor and that of the recipient and because donor oocytes are much more scarce than donor sperm, use of donor embryos seems to offer a logical means to overcome these obstacles. Technologic advances in cryopreservation have made donation of embryos a practical approach. Potential sources of donor oocytes are listed in Table 14-3.

**Pre-embryo Donation**

Donor pre-embryos may be available from donated oocytes fertilized with the husband's sperm or from excess fertilized oocytes obtained during IVF cycles. In either instance, cryopreservation avoids the need for careful coordination of donor and recipient cycles, as required whenever donor oocytes are used. Cryopreservation also enables placement of the pre-embryo during a natural cycle. Concerns over the introduction of a third party into conception and childbearing have already been discussed with regard to AID, and similar concerns apply to pre-embryo donation. IVF using donor oocytes or donor pre-embryos, however, raises additional serious questions regarding compensation for the donor, surgical risks, and as yet unresolved legal issues with regard to pre-embryo custodianship. These concerns are tabulated in Table 14-4.

**Table 14-4. Concerns regarding donor oocytes and donor pre-embryos**

Surgical risks to donor if donation is the prime intent of the procedure
Possible transmission of a genetic disorder
Potential for consanguinity
Introduction of a third party into the marital unit
Psychological effects of asymmetric parenthood in the case of donor oocytes
Ethical concerns regarding third-party gametes and lack of genetic link to parents
    in the case of donor pre-embryos
Immunologic rejection
Legal issues
Compensation for the donor

## Cryopreservation

Successful cryopreservation of pre-embryos has added new dimensions to IVF programs. One of the significant benefits is that it permits all oocytes to be retrieved and inseminated after stimulation, with storage for subsequent use of embryos obtained in excess of those required for replacement. This flexibility alleviates the frustration and dilemmas regarding the disposition of excess fertilized oocytes. By providing more pre-embryos for later transfer, cryopreservation accomplishes several important objectives: It reduces the need for subsequent surgical procedures to acquire oocytes; enables replacement during a natural cycle; theoretically leads to enhanced overall success using only a single procedure for follicle aspiration to serve as a potential reservoir for multiple individual conception cycles; and provides the flexibility of donation to others. Cryopreservation simultaneously raises a host of potential problems. Success at cryopreservation requires unique skills and experience as well as the need for specialized equipment, thus raising critical financial considerations. Questions regarding custodianship during preservation, prolonged preservation, possible posthumous transfer, and inheritance rights, are more serious in the long run. In general, cryopreservation of human pre-embryos is currently acceptable, and institutions employing this procedure have enjoyed a respectable record of resultant healthy offspring. Society's concerns are similar to those raised when IVF was first introduced, namely it represents a technologic intrusion into the natural process of reproduction. Prior to incorporation of cryopreservation within an IVF program, recruitment and training of knowledgeable, experienced counselors are mandatory to outline with the couples involved the myriad of contingencies attendant on the responsibility for gamete or pre-embryo storage.

Many parallels can be found between pre-embryo donation and organ donation. The matter of compensation of or payment to the donor is a case in point. It is customary in organ transplant programs for the recipient to accept responsibility for the costs of maintenance of the deceased and for removal of his or her organs. Likewise, because purchase or sale of an embryo is an offensive practice, appropriate policies must be established that meet both practical and societal concerns. Policies regarding duration of storage need to be resolved, including the possibility of posthumous use, the risks of death or divorce, and the woman's natural duration of reproductive capacity.

Considering that the alternative to pre-embryo transfer, disposal of pre-embryos, is also offensive, it would seem preferable to require all parents to agree to one of the two other options: transfer or donation of all pre-embryos. Furthermore, programs that utilized cryopreservation must require that the donating couple execute a form relinquishing their rights and obligations to the resultant offspring, in the event that their pre-embryo(s) are donated. The ethical and legal issues surrounding cryopreservation of human embryos have recently been reviewed (4).

## Surrogacy

Surrogacy implies substitution of a function. With respect to reproductive technology, a surrogate gestational mother who provides a uterus for gestation supplies only the gestational component of reproduction; therefore, she differs from a surrogate mother who not only substitutes for the functional deficit by lending the use of her uterus, but also provides the female gamete required for conception. Situations that require a surrogate gestational mother are relatively rare, whereas there are multiple potential applications for a surrogate mother. The surrogate mother is generally artificially inseminated with sperm from the male member of the infertile couple. On conceiving, she carries the pregnancy and is then expected to relinquish the child to the infertile couple after its birth. Since the male member of the couple is the actual father, his wife will adopt the child. Surrogate motherhood is invoked to provide the child with a genetic link to one member of the couple, the husband. Whereas in AID both the gestational and genetic links are provided by the mother and a third party donates the sperm, in surrogate motherhood the husband's sperm is used to enable conception. This step then is actually the only difference between surrogate motherhood and adoption. Surrogacy remains the most controversial of the new reproductive technologies, largely because of the surrogate's significant role in conception and the intimate nature of the bonding process during gestation and delivery. Legal issues are extensive and are currently being considered by many state legislatures as well as by ethics organizations worldwide. The American Fertility Society considers gestational surrogacy to be a clinical experiment, pending availability and evaluation of data regarding both short- and long-term consequences of the procedure. The issue of finances is not completely resolved because certain forms of compensation fall within the realm of "baby selling" laws, and yet reimbursement of expenses incurred by the surrogate does not seem at all unreasonable. Until more data are released and laws are enacted, it is safe to conclude that it is not necessarily unethical to offer surrogate arrangements to certain infertile couples. Currently, a large gap exists between supply of and demand for surrogate mothers. The screening process must be thorough and accompanied by substantiation of a composite informed consent. The surrogate must be emotionally and physically healthy. Agreements need to be carefully worded and kept on file. The willingness of a physician to provide the service or his or her wish to avoid involvement with surrogate arrangements must be honored. All programs that provide surrogate services should keep long-term records to facilitate data analysis.

Surrogacy antedates all other "new reproductive technologies" by centuries, having been practiced privately by couples since biblical times. Two surrogate cases recently became the focal point of international attention. The Baby M case in New Jersey highlights the major hazard of a surrogate arrangement, namely the ultimate desire of a surrogate mother to retain the infant she has carried for 40 weeks. The second case, in Johannesburg, South Africa, involved a woman who had previously undergone hysterectomy, but participated in IVF using her own oocytes, her husband's sperm, and her 46-year-old mother's uterus, and ultimately gave birth to triplets. Although the potential for retention of the baby by the surrogate mother was eliminated in this instance by use of a family member for this function, the hazard to fetus and mother of an older woman having a pregnancy are apparent. That a 46-year-old can carry her own grandchildren is in itself a bizarre event. Many state legislatures are currently grappling with regulation of the practice of surrogate motherhood. Some states (Louisiana, Florida, Kentucky, Michigan, and Nebraska) have banned commercial agreements or contracts. Preplanned adoption arrangements that encompass voluntary, noncommercial surrogacy remain as possibilities for the future. The major issues involving surrogate motherhood that need to be addressed are itemized in Table 14-5.

**Table 14-5. Surrogate motherhood issues that need to be addressed**

Psychological effects on all parties
Effects of bonding in utero
Appropriate screening of surrogate and sperm donor
Appropriate precautions during pregnancy
Effects of a meeting between couple and surrogate
Effects on surrogate's own family
Effects of nondisclosure on a child
Effects of surrogacy on society
Commercial aspects of surrogacy

These issues of ethical interpretation revolving around IVF and related technology have prompted worldwide evaluation. In Victoria, Australia, the Infertility (Medical Procedures) Act of Parliament placed Victoria as the first jurisdiction in the world to enact comprehensive legislation specifying what physicians and scientists may and may not do in attempting to overcome infertility.

The new legislation places control firmly in the hands of the government. Anyone carrying out human fertilization outside the body, or experimenting with human embryos, except in circumstances permitted by the law, faces a substantial fine or imprisonment for up to 4 years. Based on the recommendations of the Waller Committee, the new legislation states that

Only approved hospitals are permitted to engage in IVF and related technologies.
Only married couples will be treated (although couples in a de facto relationship who are already having treatment may remain on the IVF program).
All patients must, for at least 12 months before IVF is attempted, have sought treatment for infertility.
The use of donated sperm, eggs, or embryos is to be a last resort—permissible only when it has been established that there is no other reasonable prospect of pregnancy, or that any child the woman would have without such a donation would be likely to carry a heredity disorder.
No payment may be made for sperm, eggs, or embryos, other than a prescribed amount for travel or medical expenses incurred by the donor.
Embryo freezing is permitted, provided it is carried out with the aim of implanting the embryo at a later date.
Experiments of embryos are to be approved by a Standing Review and Advisory Committee. (Although the Waller Committee stipulated a time limit of 14 days for such experimentation, the new legislation does not). The Committee must report to the minister any experimental procedures it approves.
Commercial surrogate motherhood arrangements are prohibited; it is an offense, punishable by up to 2 years in prison, to give or receive payment for acting as a surrogate mother.
Cloning and the creation of animal-human hybrids are prohibited.

The Medical Research Council of Great Britain in 1982 set forth principles regarding research with human gametes:

1. Scientifically sound research involving experiments on the processes and products of IVF between human gametes is ethically acceptable and should be allowed to proceed on condition that there is not intent to transfer to the uterus any embryo resulting from or used in such experiments, and that the aim of the research is clearly defined and directly relevant to clinical diagnosis and treatment of infertility or inherited disease.

2. Informed consent to research involving human ova or sperm banks should be obtained in every case from the donors. Sperm from sperm banks should not be used unless preserved specifically for research purposes. Approval for each experiment should be obtained from the appropriate scientific and local ethical committees.

3. When human ova have been obtained and fertilized in vitro for a therapeutic purpose and are no longer required for that purpose, it would be ethical to use them for soundly designed research provided that the informed consent of both donors was obtained.

4. Human ova fertilized with human sperm should not be cultured in vitro beyond the implantation stage; that it should not be stored for unspecified research use.

5. Although it is not always possible to extrapolate results from animal work to the human situation, results from animal gametes and embryos are useful to elucidate the potential risk of IVF and embryo transfer. Tests of animal embryos and appropriate animal models are necessary before it can be assumed that the frozen storage of the embryo does not cause harm to the conceptus.

6. Studies on interspecies fertilization are valuable in providing information on the penetration capacity and chromosome complement of sperm from subfertile males and should be supported. The fertilized ovum should not be allowed to develop beyond the early cleavage state.

The Ethics Committee of the American Fertility Society presented its report entitled "Ethical considerations of the new reproductive technologies" in September 1986 (1). Regarding the new reproductive technologies, the Committee summarized its report as follows:

Several reproductive options now use third parties—donor sperm, donor eggs, donor pre-embryos, and the various forms of surrogacy. There is one member of the committee who finds any third party involvements ethically problematic (Appendix A).

"The Committee agrees that the basic rationale for in vitro fertilization (IVF) outweighs foreseeable risks to the potential offspring, the couple, and society. It unanimously finds that basic IVF is ethically acceptable (chapter 13).

The Committee also finds ethically acceptable the use of artificial insemination with husband's sperm (AIH) for demonstrated medical indications. The use of AIH for uncertain indications or sex selection should be regarded as a clinical experiment, rather than conventional practice (chapter 14).

The Committee finds the use of artificial insemination with donor sperm (AID) ethically acceptable (chapter 15).

Similarly, the Committee finds ethically acceptable in IVF the use of donor sperm (chapter 16), the use of donor eggs (chapter 17), and the use of donor pre-embryos (chapter 18).

The Committee finds that uterine lavage for pre-embryo transfer should be regarded as a clinical experiment, general application of which is premature (chapter 19).

The Committee finds ethically acceptable the cryopreservation of sperm (chapter 20). Further, the Committee recommends that the American Fertility Society initiate steps to establish performance standards for sperm banks.

The Committee finds that much more preliminary investigation is needed in cryopreservation of the unfertilized egg. In the event that these studies indicate that clinical application seems feasible, the application should be regarded as a clinical experiment. General application of which is premature (chapter 21).

The Committee finds that the study of cryopreservation is desirable and should be encouraged, but the Committee regards clinical programs in the cryopreservation of fertilized eggs and pre-embryos as clinical experiments, general application of which is premature (chapter 22).

The Committee finds ethically acceptable research on the pre-embryo for the purpose of generating new knowledge not otherwise obtainable for benefiting human health (chapter 23).

The Committee opposes the use of surrogate gestational mothers for nonmedical reasons. The Committee recognizes, however, that there could be a role for surrogate gestation in reproductive medicine. If surrogate gestational motherhood is used, it should be pursued as a clinical experiment. Therefore, general application of this procedure is considered to be premature (chapter 25).

The Committee is concerned about quality assurance in the use of reproductive technologies. The Committee recommends that the American Fertility Society, in conjunction with other public and professional groups, should take the initiative in stimulating active training, in reviewing standards, in providing information, and in encouraging professional and public oversight of ongoing reproductive technologies (chapter 26).

The Committee recognizes the need for continuing, comprehensive analysis of current policy to match the rapidly advancing reproductive technologies. For that reason, the Committee recommends that the initiative taken by the American Fertility Society in launching this study and report should be continued, preferably in concert with other professional groups involved in reproductive medicine. The Committee recommends that the American Fertility Society should actively seek and encourage a national effort to assess broader implications and requirements of the new technologies through one or more mechanisms at the highest level of credibility and general access. The group should consider means of implementing for any of its recommendations but should not itself be implementative in function. The Committee also recommends that the American Fertility Society promote an effort to assure wide public understanding of reproduction and its technologies as fundamental to effective reproductive policy. The Committee believes that appropriate research should be encouraged in support of the new technologies as fundamental to effective reproductive policy. To this end, the Committee recommends that the American Fertility Society should seek support within the biomedical community in an effort to persuade the Department of Health and Human Services to revise its policies and encourage funding for approved innovative reproductive research proposals (chapter 27)."

In 1987, a second Ethics Committee was convened by the American Fertility Society to address the *Instruction on the Respect for Human Life and Its Origin and on the Dignity of Procreation* issued by the Congregation for the Doctrine of the Faith. The Committee was concerned about the impact of the *Instruction* on four groups: (1) those individuals who face problems that could be resolved by new reproductive technologies; (2) those who apply these technologies; (3) those who have the responsibility for establishing institutional policies on these techniques, and (4) those who are involved in developing or influencing public policy in a legislative or regulatory manner. The following statements summarize the Committee's conclusions (2):

"The Committee reaffirmed the finding that the use of heterologous gametes is also ethically acceptable, provided that various precautions and guidelines are observed, as outlined in its previous report.

The Committee recognized and re-evaluated the long-debated and very complex issues of the moral state of the gamete, zygote, pre-embryo, embryo, and fetus. The reasons for believing that progressive development were set forth here and in the previous document. The Committee reaffirmed the position that experimentation on the pre-embryo in conformity with the policies and guidelines, as previously expressed, can be ethically justifiable and, indeed, necessary, if the human condition is to be improved.

The Committee was especially concerned lest the pluralistic nature of society be overlooked. It recognized that societal judgments about the reproductive technologies have changed and continue to change, necessitating a continuing dialogue to assure that these changes are reflected in current and future practices. For this reason, the Committee views with alarm the call for legislation based on doctrines not adequately supported by human experience or scientific data.

The Committee welcomes and encourages continued re-evaluation of the changing societal and moral issues and views involved in the ever-evolving new reproductive technologies."

## REFERENCES

1. American Fertility Society, Ethics Committee. Ethical considerations of the new reproductive technologies. *Fertil. Steril.* 46(3), 1986.
2. American Fertility Society, Ethics Committee. Instruction on the respect for human life and its origin and on the dignity of procreation. *Fertil. Steril.* 1987.
3. Ontario Law Reforms Commission. *Report on Human Artificial Reproduction and Related Matters.* Toronto: Ministry of the Attorney General, 1985.
4. Robertson, J. A. Ethical and legal issues in cryopreservation of human embryos. *Fertil. Steril.* 47:371, 1987.
5. United Kingdom, Department of Health and Society Security. *Report of the Committee of Inquiry into Human Fertilization and Embryology.* London: Her Majesty's Stationery Office, 1984.
6. Victoria Committee to Consider the Social, Ethical and Legal Issues Arising from In Vitro Fertilization. Victoria, Australia: F.D. Atkinson Government Printer, 1984.

# IVF Financial Considerations

## Marian D. Damewood and Edward E. Wallach

Many practical aspects are encountered in establishing an in vitro fertilization (IVF) program as well as before selecting the IVF procedure as a therapeutic modality. Foremost among considerations is the usefulness of the procedure itself in aiding the infertile couple. The questions that need to be addressed include the applicability of IVF and embryo transfer (ET) as a procedure for any given couple, the statistical possibilities for its success, and alternative procedures and their likelihood for success. On the other hand, economic feasibility must be considered seriously in comparing IVF-ET and reconstructive tubal surgery as therapeutic modalities. The results of therapy using IVF-ET apply only to the cycle in which the procedure is performed. In contrast, reconstructive tubal surgery may provide relatively long-term opportunities for conception following surgery; often a single reconstructive surgical procedure enables the establishment of more than one pregnancy. In situations in which other forms of therapy are not feasible, e.g., absence of both fallopian tubes, the sole considerations are (1) the availability of IVF, (2) the results of the program conducting the procedure, and (3) the cost of the procedure.

Another practical consideration in selecting a therapeutic procedure involves the extent to which a third party (medical insurance carrier) will reimburse the providers (physician[s], hospital, clinic) for diagnostic and therapeutic procedures. Included among these procedures are a host of professional, laboratory, and hospital fees. The legislature of Maryland has taken a stand (March, 1985) emphasizing to third parties providing health insurance in Maryland that IVF is a proved form of therapy for use in certain types of infertility, is no longer an experimental technique, and should be reimbursible as is any other acceptable type of infertility treatment. Appended to this chapter are

1. The economics to be considered involving start-up costs required to establish a program and the costs to the patients
2. The Blue Cross/Blue Shield statements to Johns Hopkins Hospital prior to the legislative hearings
3. A letter to the legislature by Edward E. Wallach, M.D., stressing that IVF is a widely accepted procedure and its costs should be reimbursed by Blue Cross/Blue Shield
4. A statement delivered to the legislature (March 12, 1985) by Marian D. Damewood, M.D., to the same effect
5. State of Maryland—Senate Bill No. 793
6. State of Maryland—House Bill No. 1660

## REFERENCE

1. Dandekar, P. V., and Quigley, M. M. Laboratory set-up for human in vitro fertilization. *Fertil. Steril.* 42:1, 1984.

# Appendix 15-1. Economics to be Considered*

1. Estimated Start-Up Costs for Program
   a. Equipment and supplies _____
   b. Reproductive endocrinologist(s) (partial) _____
   c. Laboratory staff _____
   d. Nurse coordinator _____
   e. Secretary _____
   f. Additional IVF technical help _____
   Total Program Expense
2. Patient Expenses
   a. *Ovulation Induction Phase*
      (1) Mouse embryo culture _____
      (2) Ultrasonography (prof. fee) _____
      (3) Ultrasonography (hospital) _____
      (4) Laboratory medicine (assays) _____
      (5) Reproductive endocrine fees _____
      Total _____
   b. *Laparoscopy Phase*
      (1) Reproductive endocrinology (prof. fee) _____
      (2) Anesthesiology (prof. fee) _____
      (3) Operating room (hospital) _____
      (4) Recovery room (hospital) _____
      (5) Anesthesia (hospital) _____
   c. *Andrology*
      (1) Andrology laboratory fees _____
      Total _____
   d. *In Vitro Fertilization Laboratory Phase*
      (1) Laboratory Staff _____
   e. *Embryo Transfer Phase*
      (1) Laboratory Staff (prof. fee) _____
      (2) Hospital fee _____
      Total _____
Grand Total Patient Expenses _____

*The figures have purposely been omitted because of changes in costs over time.

164

# Appendix 15-2. Blue Cross/Blue Shield Rebuttal Reasons for which In Vitro Fertilization is Considered Investigative/Experimental

1. The rate at which pregnancy is achieved to the period of viability is less among in vitro patients than it is among those conceiving naturally.
2. Little is known about the long term effects or the incidence of abnormal pregnancy among those who undergo in vitro fertilization; in fact, in vitro fertilization is used in the research field to learn how genetic defects arise and are transmitted and how they might be prevented or treated.
3. The process called in vitro fertilization does not directly treat or attempt to treat a pathological problem, rather it circumvents the pathology altogether.
4. In vitro fertilization is purely an elective procedure which is never performed as a means to sustain life or prevent death, promote longevity or health, or delay/prevent/palliate illness.
5. In vitro fertilization is not a standard and accepted treatment for fertilization in that it is not widely/readily available to the population requiring such attention. The procedure requires special expertise on the part of the physician and other support personnel and the use of sophisticated equipment.

# Appendix 15-3.  Excerpts from Letter by Edward E. Wallach, M.D.

. . . In Vitro Fertilization is a vital series of procedures which have aided considerably in the successful care of infertile couples. I consider it a well-established clinical procedure with a 7 year history of success and refinements in technique. As such, it is my belief that no insurance carrier should exclude in vitro fertilization from its benefits.

# Appendix 15-4. Statement Delivered by Marian Damewood, M.D.

My name is Dr. Marian Damewood. I am Assistant Professor of Gynecology/Obstetrics at the Johns Hopkins Hospital. I am the Director of the In Vitro Fertilization Program at Johns Hopkins. I'd first like to note that I personally support Bill No. 1660, and I have had the opportunity to work with many of the patients that are here in this room today. I'd like to enlist your support for this bill without which many patients such as these would have no opportunity to enter an IVF program. *A comment on the contention that in vitro fertilization is considered investigational or experimental:*

At present as of the 1984 World Congress of Human Reproduction and present statistics, over 1,000 babies have been born as a result of this established procedure. Over 200 new centers for in vitro fertilization are open or are to open in 1984–85, with over 70 centers in full operation for greater than 1 year. Thirty-five percent of these centers are operating for 4 or more years.

*A comment on the rate at which pregnancy is achieved to the period of viability being less than those conceiving naturally:*

1. Natural conception rate with 1 month of attempt of a couple is approximately 25%.
2. The average conception rate with 1 month of attempt in in vitro fertilization is 20% to 25%. I'd like to note also that in some areas of contention it has been noted that the miscarriage rate is higher than the general population. The miscarriage rate in the general population is 20%. The miscarriage rate in in vitro fertilization programs is similar and may seem higher due to the early detection of very early miscarriages in carefully monitored in vitro fertilization patients.

*A comment on the contention that little is known regarding long-term effects on IVF children:*

As of the 1984 World Congress over 1000 babies have been born as of results of in vitro fertilization. Four of these infants had congenital anomalies. This represents a rate of congenital anomaly which is less than that of the general population.

*A comment on the contention that the process does not treat or attempt to treat pathology while it circumvents pathology all together:*

Essentially in vitro fertilization is offered to those patients with end stage intractable infertility. Endometriosis, tubal disease and sperm problems have already been treated to the best of medical knowledge with surgery or medication prior to entering a patient into the in vitro program.

*A comment on the fact that in vitro fertilization is an elective procedure and is not a life or death situation:*

Many surgical procedures are elective and this particular process is performed as a means to aid in conception to bring life into the world for couples desiring a child of their own. It must be emphasized that other less costly procedures are done first prior to in vitro fertilization.

*A comment on the contention that in vitro fertilization is not readily available:*

As noted there are 200 centers at present operating. There are two in the Baltimore area. In vitro fertilization does not require sophisticated equipment or unusual expertise in this area. A gynecologist experienced in laparoscopy and ovulation induction as well as the standard hospital laboratory and equipment is all that is required. It is not experimental. It has been proven as therapy for intractable infertility and is essentially the last hope for a couple desiring a biologic off-spring.

# Appendix 15-5.  Senate Bill No. 793 (5lr3381)

Introduced by Senator Clark

Read and Examined by Proofreader:

_____

Proofreader.

_____

Proofreader.

Sealed with the Great Seal and presented to the Governor, for his approval this_____ day of_____ at_____ o'clock,_____M.

_____

President.

CHAPTER _____

1   AN ACT concerning

2          Insurance - In Vitro Fertilization

3   FOR-the-purpose-of-requiring-that-each--health--insurance--policy
4       certificate-or-contract-issued-in-the-State-include-benefits
5       for--inpatient-and-outpatient-expenses-arising-from-in-vitro
6       fertilization---procedures---performed---on---the----policy,
7       certificate,--or--contract--holder-or-the-holder's-dependent
8       spouse certain-contracts-issued-by-nonprofit-health--service
9       plans--and-policies-issued-by-insurance-companies-to-provide
10      benefits-for-expenses-arising-from--in--vitro--fertilization
11      procedures-performed-on-certain-covered-individuals-or-their
12      dependent-spouses.
13  FOR the purpose of prohibiting the exclusion in certain group or
14      individual contracts or certificates issued or delivered  by
15      nonprofit  health  service  plans  and  policies  issued  or
16      delivered   by  insurance  companies  of  all  benefits  for
17      expenses arising  from  in  vitro  fertilization  procedures
18      performed  on certain covered individuals or their dependent
19      spouses; requiring that benefits for in vitro  fertilization
20      be  provided  to  the  same  extent as benefits provided for
21      other    pregnancy-related    procedures    under    certain

------------------------------------------------------------------

EXPLANATION: CAPITALS INDICATE MATTER ADDED TO EXISTING LAW.
    [Brackets] indicate matter deleted from existing law.
    Underlining indicates amendments to bill.
    Strike-out indicates matter stricken from the bill by
    amendment or deleted from the law by amendment.

2                    SENATE BILL No. 793

1  circumstances; and generally relating  to  benefits  for  in
2  vitro fertilization.

3  BY adding to

4       Article 48A - Insurance Code
5       Section 354CC, 470V, and 477CC
6       Annotated Code of Maryland
7       (1979 Replacement Volume and 1984 Supplement)

8       SECTION  1.  BE  IT  ENACTED  BY  THE  GENERAL  ASSEMBLY  OF
9  MARYLAND, That the Laws of Maryland read as follows:

10                    Article 48A - Insurance Code

11  354CC.

12  ~~EACH--GROUP-MEDICAL-OR-MAJOR-MEDICAL-CONTRACT-OR-CERTIFICATE~~
13  ~~ISSUED-OR-DELIVERED--WITHIN--THE--STATE--BY--A--NONPROFIT--HEALTH~~
14  ~~SERVICE--PLAN--SHALL-INCLUDE-BENEFITS-FOR-INPATIENT-OR-OUTPATIENT~~
15  ~~EXPENSES-ARISING-FROM-IN-VITRO-FERTILIZATION-PROCEDURES-PERFORMED~~
16  ~~ON-THE-SUBSCRIBER-OR-THE-SUBSCRIBER'S-DEPENDENT-SPOUSE.~~

17  ~~EVERY-INDIVIDUAL-OR-GROUP-CONTRACT-DELIVERED-OR--ISSUED--FOR~~
18  ~~DELIVERY--IN--THIS-STATE-ON-AN-EXPENSE-INCURRED-BASIS-UNDER-WHICH~~
19  ~~MATERNITY--BENEFITS--ARE--PROVIDED--FOR--EXPENSES--ARISING---FROM~~
20  ~~PREGNANCY--AND--CHILDBIRTH--SHALL--PROVIDE--BENEFITS-FOR-EXPENSES~~
21  ~~ARISING-FROM-IN-VITRO-FERTILIZATION-PROCEDURES-PERFORMED-ON.~~

22           ~~(1)--THE-SUBSCRIBER;-OR~~

23           ~~(2)--THE-DEPENDENT-SPOUSE-OF--THE--SUBSCRIBER--IF--THE~~
24  ~~CONTRACT-OTHERWISE-COVERS-THE-DEPENDENT-SPOUSE.~~

25       EACH   GROUP   OR INDIVIDUAL MEDICAL OR MAJOR MEDICAL CONTRACT
26  OR  CERTIFICATE  ISSUED  OR  DELIVERED  WITHIN  THE  STATE  BY  A
27  NONPROFIT   HEALTH   SERVICE   PLAN   AND   WHICH   PROVIDES
28  PREGNANCY-RELATED  BENEFITS,  MAY  NOT  EXCLUDE  BENEFITS FOR ALL
29  OUTPATIENT  EXPENSES  ARISING  FROM  IN  VITRO  FERTILIZATION
30  PROCEDURES  PERFORMED  ON  THE  SUBSCRIBER  OR  THE  SUBSCRIBER'S
31  DEPENDENT SPOUSE, PROVIDED THAT:

32           (1)  BENEFITS  UNDER THIS SECTION SHALL BE PROVIDED TO
33  THE  SAME  EXTENT  AS  THE  BENEFITS  PROVIDED  FOR  OTHER
34  PREGNANCY-RELATED PROCEDURES;

35           (2)  THE  PATIENT IS A SUBSCRIBER OR COVERED DEPENDENT
36  OF THE SUBSCRIBER;

37           (3)  THE PATIENT'S OOCYTES  ARE  FERTILIZED  WITH  THE
38  PATIENT'S SPOUSE'S SPERM;

39           (4) (I)  THE  PATIENT  AND THE PATIENT'S SPOUSE HAVE A
40  HISTORY OF INFERTILITY OF AT LEAST 5 YEARS' DURATION; OR

SENATE BILL No. 793                                    3

1   (II)  THE INFERTILITY IS ASSOCIATED WITH 1 OR
2   MORE OF THE FOLLOWING MEDICAL CONDITIONS:

3                    1.  ENDOMETRIOSIS;

4                    2.  EXPOSURE     IN     UTERO     TO
5   DIETHYLSTILBESTROL, COMMONLY KNOWN AS DES; OR

6                    3.  BLOCKAGE OF, OR SURGICAL REMOVAL OF, 1
7   OR BOTH FALLOPIAN TUBES (LATERAL OR BILATERAL SALPINGECTOMY);

8          (5)  THE    PATIENT   HAS   BEEN  UNABLE  TO  ATTAIN  A
9   SUCCESSFUL  PREGNANCY  THROUGH   ANY   LESS   COSTLY   APPLICABLE
10  INFERTILITY  TREATMENTS FOR WHICH COVERAGE IS AVAILABLE UNDER THE
11  CONTRACT OR CERTIFICATION; AND

12         (6)  THE  IN  VITRO  FERTILIZATION  PROCEDURES   ARE
13  PERFORMED  AT  MEDICAL  FACILITIES  THAT  CONFORM TO THE AMERICAN
14  COLLEGE OF OBSTETRIC  AND  GYNECOLOGY  GUIDELINES  FOR  IN  VITRO
15  FERTILIZATION  CLINICS  OR  TO  THE  AMERICAN  FERTILITY  SOCIETY
16  MINIMAL STANDARDS FOR PROGRAMS OF IN VITRO FERTILIZATION.

17  470V.

18     ~~EACH--HOSPITAL--OR-MAJOR-MEDICAL-INSURANCE-POLICY-WRITTEN-ON~~
19  ~~AN-EXPENSE-INCURRED-BASIS,--WHICH--IS--DELIVERED--OR--ISSUED--FOR~~
20  ~~DELIVERY--IN--THE--STATE,-SHALL-INCLUDE-BENEFITS-FOR-INPATIENT-OR~~
21  ~~OUTPATIENT--EXPENSES--ARISING---FROM---IN---VITRO---FERTILIZATION~~
22  ~~PROCEDURES--PERFORMED-ON-THE-POLICY-HOLDER-OR-THE-POLICY-HOLDER'S~~
23  ~~DEPENDENT-SPOUSE.~~

24     ~~EVERY-INDIVIDUAL-POLICY-OF--HOSPITAL--OR--MEDICAL--INSURANCE~~
25  ~~DELIVERED--OR--ISSUED--FOR--DELIVERY--IN-THIS-STATE-ON-AN-EXPENSE~~
26  ~~INCURRED-BASIS-UNDER-WHICH-MATERNITY-BENEFITS--ARE--PROVIDED--FOR~~
27  ~~EXPENSES--ARISING--FROM--PREGNANCY--AND--CHILDBIRTH-SHALL-PROVIDE~~
28  ~~BENEFITS--FOR--EXPENSES--ARISING--FROM--IN--VITRO---FERTILIZATION~~
29  ~~PROCEDURES-PERFORMED-ON:~~

30         ~~(1)--THE-POLICYHOLDER,-OR~~

31         ~~(2)--THE--DEPENDENT--SPOUSE-OF-THE-POLICYHOLDER-IF-THE~~
32  ~~POLICY-OTHERWISE-COVERS-THE-DEPENDENT-SPOUSE.~~

33     EACH HOSPITAL OR MAJOR MEDICAL INSURANCE POLICY  WRITTEN  ON
34  AN  EXPENSE  INCURRED  BASIS,  WHICH  IS  DELIVERED OR ISSUED FOR
35  DELIVERY IN  THE  STATE,  AND  WHICH  PROVIDES  PREGNANCY-RELATED
36  BENEFITS,  MAY  NOT  EXCLUDE BENEFITS FOR ALL OUTPATIENT EXPENSES
37  ARISING FROM IN VITRO FERTILIZATION PROCEDURES PERFORMED  ON  THE
38  POLICYHOLDER  OR  THE  POLICYHOLDER'S  DEPENDENT SPOUSE, PROVIDED
39  THAT:

40         (1)  BENEFITS UNDER THIS SECTION SHALL BE PROVIDED  TO
41  THE  SAME EXTENT AS BENEFITS PROVIDED FOR OTHER PREGNANCY-RELATED
42  PROCEDURES;

4                        SENATE BILL No. 793

1       (2) THE PATIENT IS A POLICYHOLDER OR COVERED
2   DEPENDENT OF THE POLICYHOLDER;

3       (3) THE PATIENT'S OOCYTES ARE FERTILIZED WITH THE
4   PATIENT'S SPOUSE'S SPERM;

5       (4) (I) THE PATIENT AND THE PATIENT'S SPOUSE HAVE A
6   HISTORY OF INFERTILITY OF AT LEAST 5 YEARS' DURATION; OR

7       (II) THE INFERTILITY IS ASSOCIATED WITH 1 OR
8   MORE OF THE FOLLOWING MEDICAL CONDITIONS:

9       1.  ENDOMETRIOSIS;

10      2.  EXPOSURE IN UTERO TO
11  DIETHYLSTILBESTROL, COMMONLY KNOWN AS DES; OR

12      3.  BLOCKAGE OF, OR SURGICAL REMOVAL OF, 1
13  OR BOTH FALLOPIAN TUBES (LATERAL OR BILATERAL SALPINGECTOMY);

14      (5) THE PATIENT HAS BEEN UNABLE TO ATTAIN A
15  SUCCESSFUL PREGNANCY THROUGH ANY LESS COSTLY APPLICABLE
16  INFERTILITY TREATMENTS FOR WHICH COVERAGE IS AVAILABLE UNDER THE
17  POLICY; AND

18      (6) THE IN VITRO FERTILIZATION PROCEDURES ARE
19  PERFORMED AT MEDICAL FACILITIES THAT CONFORM TO THE AMERICAN
20  COLLEGE OF OBSTETRIC AND GYNECOLOGY GUIDELINES FOR IN VITRO
21  FERTILIZATION CLINICS OR TO THE AMERICAN FERTILITY SOCIETY
22  MINIMAL STANDARDS FOR PROGRAMS OF IN VITRO FERTILIZATION.

23  477CC.

24  EACH-GROUP-OR-BLANKET--HEALTH--INSURANCE--POLICY--ISSUED--OR
25  DELIVERED--WITHIN--THE--STATE--ON-AN-EXPENSE-INCURRED-BASIS-SHALL
26  INCLUDE-BENEFITS-FOR-INPATIENT--OR--OUTPATIENT--EXPENSES--ARISING
27  FROM---IN---VITRO---FERTILIZATION--PROCEDURES--PERFORMED--ON--THE
28  CERTIFICATE-HOLDER-OR-THE-CERTIFICATE-HOLDER'S-DEPENDENT-SPOUSE.

29  EVERY-GROUP-OR-BLANKET-HEALTH-INSURANCE-POLICY-DELIVERED--OR
30  ISSUED--FOR--DELIVERY--IN-THIS-STATE-ON-AN-EXPENSE-INCURRED-BASIS
31  UNDER-WHICH-MATERNITY-BENEFITS-ARE-PROVIDED-FOR-EXPENSES--ARISING
32  FROM-PREGNANCY-AND-CHILDBIRTH-SHALL-PROVIDE-BENEFITS-FOR-EXPENSES
33  ARISING-FROM-IN-VITRO-FERTILIZATION-PROCEDURES-PERFORMED-ON.

34  (1)--ANY-COVERED-EMPLOYEE-OR-COVERED-MEMBER;-OR

35  (2)--ANY--DEPENDENT--SPOUSE--OF--A-COVERED-EMPLOYEE-OR
36  COVERED-MEMBER-IF--THE--POLICY--OTHERWISE--COVERS--THE--DEPENDENT
37  SPOUSE.

38  EACH GROUP OR BLANKET HEALTH INSURANCE POLICY ISSUED OR
39  DELIVERED WITHIN THE STATE ON AN EXPENSE INCURRED BASIS AND WHICH
40  PROVIDES PREGNANCY-RELATED BENEFITS, MAY NOT EXCLUDE BENEFITS FOR
41  ALL OUTPATIENT EXPENSES ARISING FROM IN VITRO FERTILIZATION

SENATE BILL No. 793                                    5

1  PROCEDURES PERFORMED ON THE CERTIFICATE HOLDER OR THE CERTIFICATE
2  HOLDER'S DEPENDENT SPOUSE, PROVIDED THAT:

3          (1)  BENEFITS  UNDER THIS SECTION SHALL BE PROVIDED TO
4  THE  SAME   EXTENT   AS   THE   BENEFITS   PROVIDED   FOR   OTHER
5  PREGNANCY-RELATED PROCEDURES;

6          (2)  THE  PATIENT  IS  A CERTIFICATE HOLDER OR COVERED
7  DEPENDENT OF THE CERTIFICATE HOLDER;

8          (3)  THE PATIENT'S OOCYTES  ARE  FERTILIZED  WITH  THE
9  PATIENT'S SPOUSE'S SPERM;

10         (4) (I)  THE  PATIENT  AND THE PATIENT'S SPOUSE HAVE A
11 HISTORY OF INFERTILITY OF AT LEAST 5 YEARS' DURATION; OR

12         (II)  THE INFERTILITY IS ASSOCIATED  WITH  1  OR
13 MORE OF THE FOLLOWING MEDICAL CONDITIONS:

14              1.  ENDOMETRIOSIS;

15              2.  EXPOSURE     IN     UTERO     TO
16 DIETHYLSTILBESTROL, COMMONLY KNOWN AS DES; OR

17              3.  BLOCKAGE OF, OR SURGICAL REMOVAL OF, 1
18 OR BOTH FALLOPIAN TUBES (LATERAL OR BILATERAL SALPINGECTOMY);

19         (5)  THE  PATIENT  HAS  BEEN  UNABLE  TO  ATTAIN  A
20 SUCCESSFUL  PREGNANCY  THROUGH  ANY  LESS  COSTLY  APPLICABLE
21 INFERTILITY  TREATMENTS FOR WHICH COVERAGE IS AVAILABLE UNDER THE
22 POLICY; AND

23         (6)  THE  IN  VITRO  FERTILIZATION  PROCEDURES  ARE
24 PERFORMED  AT  MEDICAL  FACILITIES  THAT  CONFORM TO THE AMERICAN
25 COLLEGE OF OBSTETRIC  AND  GYNECOLOGY  GUIDELINES  FOR  IN  VITRO
26 FERTILIZATION  CLINICS  OR  TO  THE  AMERICAN  FERTILITY  SOCIETY
27 MINIMAL STANDARDS FOR PROGRAMS OF IN VITRO FERTILIZATION.

28     SECTION  2.  AND BE IT FURTHER ENACTED, That this Act  shall
29 take effect July 1, 1985.

Approved:

_____
                                    Governor.

_____
                        President of the Senate.

_____
                    Speaker of the House of Delegates.

# Appendix 15-6. House Bill No. 1660 (5lr3418)

Introduced by Delegate Chasnoff (By Request)

Read and Examined by Proofreader:

_____

Proofreader.

_____

Proofreader.

Sealed with the Great Seal and presented to the Governor, for his approval this_____ day of_____ at_____o'clock,_____M.

_____

Speaker.

CHAPTER _____

1    AN ACT concerning

2              Insurance - In Vitro Fertilization

3    FOR-the-purpose-of requiring-that-each providing--that--a health
4    insurance-policy-certificate-or-contract-issued-in-the-State
5    include may--not--exclude benefits--for inpatient-and all
6    outpatient-expenses--arising--from--in--vitro--fertilization
7    procedures-performed-on-the-policy,-certificate,-or-contract
8    holder--or--the--holder's--dependent--spouse,-and-specifying
9    certain-restrictions-on-the-provision-;-

10   FOR the purpose of prohibiting the exclusion in certain group or
11   individual contracts or certificates issued or delivered by
12   nonprofit health service plans and policies issued or
13   delivered by insurance companies ·of all benefits for
14   expenses arising from in vitro fertilization procedures
15   performed on certain covered individuals or their dependent
16   spouses; requiring that benefits for in vitro fertilization
17   be provided to the same extent as benefits provided for
18   other pregnancy-related procedures under certain
19   circumstances; and generally relating to benefits for in
20   vitro fertilization.

-------------------------------------------------------------------
EXPLANATION: CAPITALS INDICATE MATTER ADDED TO EXISTING LAW.
    [Brackets] indicate matter deleted from existing law.
    Underlining indicates amendments to bill.
    Strike-out indicates matter stricken from the bill by
    amendment or deleted from the law by amendment.

2                          HOUSE BILL No. 1660

1   BY adding to

        Article 48A - Insurance Code
3       Section 354CC, 470V, and 477CC
4       Annotated Code of Maryland
5       (1979 Replacement Volume and 1984 Supplement)


6       SECTION 1.  BE IT ENACTED BY THE GENERAL ASSEMBLY OF
7   MARYLAND, That the Laws of Maryland read as follows:

8                       Article 48A - Insurance Code

9   354CC.

10      EACH GROUP OR INDIVIDUAL MEDICAL OR MAJOR MEDICAL CONTRACT
11  OR CERTIFICATE ISSUED OR DELIVERED WITHIN THE STATE BY A
12  NONPROFIT HEALTH SERVICE PLAN AND WHICH PROVIDES
13  PREGNANCY-RELATED BENEFITS, ~~SHALL--INCLUDE~~ MAY NOT EXCLUDE
14  BENEFITS FOR ~~INPATIENT-OR~~ ALL OUTPATIENT EXPENSES ARISING FROM IN
15  VITRO FERTILIZATION PROCEDURES PERFORMED ON THE SUBSCRIBER OR THE
16  SUBSCRIBER'S DEPENDENT SPOUSE, PROVIDED THAT:

17          (1) BENEFITS UNDER THIS SECTION SHALL BE PROVIDED TO
18  THE SAME EXTENT AS THE BENEFITS PROVIDED FOR OTHER
19  PREGNANCY-RELATED PROCEDURES;

20          ~~(1)~~ (2) THE PATIENT IS A SUBSCRIBER OR COVERED
21  DEPENDENT OF THE SUBSCRIBER;

22          ~~(2)~~ (3) THE PATIENT'S OOCYTES ARE FERTILIZED WITH THE
23  PATIENT'S SPOUSE'S SPERM;

24          ~~(3)~~ (4) (I) THE PATIENT AND THE PATIENT'S SPOUSE HAVE
25  A HISTORY OF INFERTILITY OF AT LEAST 5 YEARS' DURATION; OR

26              (II) THE INFERTILITY IS ASSOCIATED WITH ONE OR
27  MORE OF THE FOLLOWING MEDICAL CONDITIONS:

28              1.  ENDOMETRIOSIS;

29              2.  EXPOSURE IN UTERO TO
30  DIETHYLSTILBESTROL, COMMONLY KNOWN AS DES; OR

31              3.  BLOCKAGE OF, OR SURGICAL REMOVAL OF,
32  ONE OR BOTH FALLOPIAN TUBES (LATERAL OR BILATERAL ~~SALPHINGECTOMY~~
33  SALPINGECTOMY);

34          ~~(4)~~ (5) THE PATIENT HAS BEEN UNABLE TO ATTAIN A
35  SUCCESSFUL PREGNANCY THROUGH ANY LESS COSTLY APPLICABLE
36  INFERTILITY TREATMENTS FOR WHICH COVERAGE IS AVAILABLE UNDER THE
37  CONTRACT OR CERTIFICATION; AND

38          ~~(5)~~ (6) THE IN VITRO FERTILIZATION PROCEDURES ARE
39  PERFORMED AT MEDICAL FACILITIES THAT CONFORM TO THE AMERICAN
40  COLLEGE OF OBSTETRIC AND GYNECOLOGY GUIDELINES FOR IN VITRO

HOUSE BILL No. 1660                     3

1  FERTILIZATION CLINICS OR TO THE AMERICAN FERTILITY SOCIETY
2  MINIMAL STANDARDS FOR PROGRAMS OF IN VITRO FERTILIZATION.

3  470V.

4      EACH HOSPITAL OR MAJOR MEDICAL INSURANCE POLICY WRITTEN ON
5  AN EXPENSE INCURRED BASIS, WHICH IS DELIVERED OR ISSUED FOR
6  DELIVERY IN THE STATE, AND WHICH PROVIDES PREGNANCY-RELATED
7  BENEFITS, SHALL INCLUDE MAY NOT EXCLUDE BENEFITS FOR INPATIENT OR
8  ALL OUTPATIENT EXPENSES ARISING FROM IN VITRO FERTILIZATION
9  PROCEDURES PERFORMED ON THE POLICY HOLDER OR THE POLICY HOLDER'S
10 DEPENDENT SPOUSE, PROVIDED THAT:

11      (1) BENEFITS UNDER THIS SECTION SHALL BE PROVIDED TO
12 THE SAME EXTENT AS BENEFITS PROVIDED FOR OTHER PREGNANCY-RELATED
13 PROCEDURES;

14      (1) (2) THE PATIENT IS A SUBSCRIBER POLICYHOLDER OR
15 COVERED DEPENDENT OF THE SUBSCRIBER POLICYHOLDER;

16      (2) (3) THE PATIENT'S OOCYTES ARE FERTILIZED WITH THE
17 PATIENT'S SPOUSE'S SPERM;

18      (3) (4) (I) THE PATIENT AND THE PATIENT'S SPOUSE HAVE
19 A HISTORY OF INFERTILITY OF AT LEAST 5 YEARS' DURATION; OR

20      (II) THE INFERTILITY IS ASSOCIATED WITH ONE OR
21 MORE OF THE FOLLOWING MEDICAL CONDITIONS:

22          1. ENDOMETRIOSIS;

23          2. EXPOSURE IN UTERO TO
24 DIETHYLSTILBESTROL, COMMONLY KNOWN AS DES; OR

25          3. BLOCKAGE OF, OR SURGICAL REMOVAL OF,
26 ONE OR BOTH FALLOPIAN TUBES (LATERAL OR BILATERAL SALPHINGECTOMY
27 SALPINGECTOMY);

28      (4) (5) THE PATIENT HAS BEEN UNABLE TO ATTAIN A
29 SUCCESSFUL PREGNANCY THROUGH ANY LESS COSTLY APPLICABLE
30 INFERTILITY TREATMENTS FOR WHICH COVERAGE IS AVAILABLE UNDER THE
31 CONTRACT OR CERTIFICATION POLICY; AND

32      (5) (6) THE IN VITRO FERTILIZATION PROCEDURES ARE
33 PERFORMED AT MEDICAL FACILITIES THAT CONFORM TO THE AMERICAN
34 COLLEGE OF OBSTETRIC AND GYNECOLOGY GUIDELINES FOR IN VITRO
35 FERTILIZATION CLINICS OR TO THE AMERICAN FERTILITY SOCIETY
36 MINIMAL STANDARDS FOR PROGRAMS OF IN VITRO FERTILIZATION.

37 477CC.

38      EACH GROUP OR BLANKET HEALTH INSURANCE POLICY ISSUED OR
39 DELIVERED WITHIN THE STATE ON AN EXPENSE INCURRED BASIS AND WHICH
40 PROVIDES PREGNANCY-RELATED BENEFITS, SHALL INCLUDE MAY NOT
41 EXCLUDE BENEFITS FOR INPATIENT OR ALL OUTPATIENT EXPENSES ARISING
42 FROM IN VITRO FERTILIZATION PROCEDURES PERFORMED ON THE

4                          HOUSE BILL No. 1660

1  CERTIFICATE HOLDER OR THE CERTIFICATE HOLDER'S DEPENDENT  SPOUSE,
2  PROVIDED THAT:

3           (1) `BENEFITS  UNDER THIS SECTION SHALL BE PROVIDED TO
4  THE  SAME·  EXTENT  AS  THE  BENEFITS  PROVIDED  FOR  OTHER
5  PREGNANCY-RELATED PROCEDURES;

6           ~~(1)~~ (2) THE  PATIENT  IS  A  ~~SUBSCRIBER~~ CERTIFICATE
7  HOLDER OR COVERED DEPENDENT OF THE ~~SUBSCRIBER~~ CERTIFICATE HOLDER;

8           ~~(2)~~ (3) THE PATIENT'S OOCYTES ARE FERTILIZED WITH THE
9  PATIENT'S SPOUSE'S SPERM;

10          ~~(3)~~ (4) (I)  THE PATIENT AND THE PATIENT'S SPOUSE HAVE
11  A HISTORY OF INFERTILITY OF AT LEAST 5 YEARS' DURATION; OR

12          (II)  THE  INFERTILITY IS ASSOCIATED WITH ONE OR
13  MORE OF THE FOLLOWING MEDICAL CONDITIONS:

14          1.  ENDOMETRIOSIS;

15          2.  EXPOSURE  IN  UTERO  TO
16  DIETHYLSTILBESTROL, COMMONLY KNOWN AS DES; OR

17          3.  BLOCKAGE OF, OR SURGICAL  REMOVAL  OF,
18  ONE  OR BOTH FALLOPIAN TUBES (LATERAL OR BILATERAL ~~SALPHINGECTOMY~~
19  SALPINGECTOMY);

20          ~~(4)~~ (5) THE PATIENT HAS BEEN UNABLE TO ATTAIN A
21  SUCCESSFUL  PREGNANCY  THROUGH  ANY  LESS  COSTLY  APPLICABLE
22  INFERTILITY TREATMENTS FOR ·WHICH COVERAGE IS AVAILABLE UNDER  THE
23  ~~CONTRACT OR CERTIFICATION~~ POLICY; AND

24          ~~(5)~~ (6) THE  IN VITRO  FERTILIZATION PROCEDURES ARE
25  PERFORMED AT MEDICAL FACILITIES  THAT  CONFORM  TO  THE  AMERICAN
26  COLLEGE OF  OBSTETRIC  AND  GYNECOLOGY  GUIDELINES  FOR IN VITRO
27  FERTILIZATION  CLINICS  OR  TO  THE  AMERICAN  FERTILITY  SOCIETY
28  MINIMAL STANDARDS FOR PROGRAMS OF IN VITRO FERTILIZATION.

29      SECTION 2.  AND BE IT FURTHER ENACTED, That this Act  shall
30  take effect July 1, 1985.


Approved:

_____

                                    Governor.

_____

                    Speaker of the House of Delegates.

_____

                    President of the Senate.

# Index

# Index

Abortion, spontaneous
  vs. general population, 167
  with GIFT, 131
  with ovulation induction, 67, 74, 83
Acceptance into program, psychological issues with, 28
Age, of patient, 10, 11
AID (artificial insemination with donor sperm), ethics of, 155–156
AIH (artificial insemination with husband sperm), ethics of, 155
American Fertility Society, Ethics Committee of, 160–162
American Society of Psychosomatic Obstetrics and Gynecology, 32
Androgenesis, 121
Antisperm antibodies, 8, 15–16, 20–21
Application, 43, 44
Application process, IVF team during, 39
Artificial insemination with donor sperm (AID), ethics of, 155–156
Artificial insemination with husband sperm (AIH), ethics of, 155
Asthenospermia, 18–20
Autoimmunity, 8, 15–16, 20–21
Autonomy, 152
Azoospermia, 15

Beneficence, 152
Biocool freezing machine, 145
Birth defects
  vs. general population, 167
  with GIFT, 131
  with IVF, 55, 56
Blastocysts, cryopreservation of, 147
Blastomeres, 116
Blood test, 46
Blue Cross/Blue Shield, IVF-ET policy of, 165
Brief Symptom Inventory (BSI), 35
Burnout, 35

CC. See Clomiphene citrate (CC, Clomid, Serophene)
Cervical factor infertility, 8
Cleavage, process of, 116–119
Cleaving embryo, cryopreservation of, 148
Clomiphene citrate (CC, Clomid, Serophene)
  follicular maturation with, 70, 73
  hMG with, 67
  LH surge with, 76–77
  luteal phase deficiency with, 79–80
  in ovulation induction, 66
  regimens for, 79
Competitiveness, 31
Consent forms, 51–58
Coordinator, 39–42, 43
Corona radiata, 114, 115
Corpus luteum formation, 65

Cost. See Financial considerations
Cryomed freezing machine, 145
Cryopreservation
  background of, 142
  of blastocyst, 147
  of cleaving embryo, 148
  consent form for, 57–58
  cryoprotectants for, 142, 143, 144–145
  culture media for, 145
  ethics of, 157
  by fast freezing, 143–144
  freezing machines for, 145
  freezing solutions for, 147, 148
  freezing vessel for, 145
  need for, 142
  principles of, 142–144
  of pronuclear stage, 148
  protocols for, 147–148
  by rapid freezing, 144
  by slow freezing, 143–144
  storage in, 145
  thawing solutions for, 147, 148
  by vitrification, 144
Cryoprotectants, 142, 143, 144–145
Culture medium
  for cryopreservation, 145
  preparation of, 104
Cumulus cells, 65
Cumulus echo, 74
Cumulus oophorus, 114, 115

Dictyate stage, 114
Dimethyl sulphoxide (DMSO), for cryopreservation, 144
Dominance, of follicle, 64–65, 70, 72
Donor insemination, ethics of, 155–156
Donor oocytes, ethics of, 156, 157
Donor pre-embryos, ethics of, 156–157
Dulbecco's phosphate buffered saline, 104

Economic considerations. See Financial considerations
Ectopic pregnancy
  with GIFT, 130–131
  as indication for IVF, 4
  with IVF, 55
Egg penetration test, 16, 21–22
Embryo transfer
  consent form for, 51, 55–56
  data sheet for, 110
  description of, 49
  IVF team during, 41–42
  laboratory procedure for, 110–111
  number of embryos transferred, 98–99
  patient protocol for, 46, 47
  problems associated with, 99
  procedure for, 97–99
  psychological issues with, 29
Emotional issues, during IVF, 27–30
Endometriosis, 5–7

Estradiol
  in follicular development, 69–70, 72,
    74–76
  in GIFT, 134
  with GnRH analog, 81–82, 84
  and hCG administration, 78
  and luteal phase deficiency, 86
Ethics, 151–152
  American Fertility Society on, 160–162
  of artificial insemination, 155–156
  of cryopreservation, 157
  framework for, 152–153
  of in vitro fertilization, 153–155
  and legislation, 159
  Medical Research Council of Great Brit-
    ain on, 159–160
  of new reproductive technologies, 152–
    153, 154
  of oocyte donation, 156
  of pre-embryo donation, 156–157
  of surrogacy, 158–159

Failure, psychological issues with, 29
Family, information shared with, 31
Fast freezing, 143–144
Fertilization
  abnormal, 119–121
  description of, 49
  laboratory evaluation of, 107–110
  oocyte at, 115–116, 117
  oocyte before, 114–115
  psychological issues with, 28–29
Financial considerations, 163
  Blue Cross/Blue Shield policy, 165
  factors considered in, 164
  of GIFT vs. IVF-ET, 128
  legislation on, 168–176
  physicians' support of insurance cover-
    age for, 166–167
Follicle stimulating hormone (FSH)
  in dominance of follicle, 64, 69–70
  with GnRH analog, 81, 82, 83, 84
  hypothalamic-pituitary influence on,
    61–62
  in intraovarian follicular regulation, 62
  midcycle surge of, 70
  in ovulation induction, 66–67
  purified urinary, 81, 85
  in recruitment of follicle, 62–63
  in selection of follicle, 69
  in two-cell theory, 80
Follicular development
  CC/hMG for, 79–81
  clinical parameters of, 76
  dominance in, 64–65, 70, 72
  estrogen measurement during, 74–76
  GnRH analog/hMG therapy for, 81–85
  graafian follicle, 62
  hCG administration for, 78–79
  luteal phase support in, 86–87
  oral contraceptives for, 81
  ovulation induction model for, 70, 72
  physiologic principles of, 62–65, 69–70,
    71
  preovulatory follicle, 62

recruitment in, 62–63, 69, 70
selection in, 63–64, 69, 70, 72
sonography of, 71–74
spontaneous LH surge with, 76–77
Freezing machines, 145
Freezing phase, 143–144
Freezing solutions, 147, 148
Freezing vessel, 145
Frozen pre-embryos. See Cryopreservation
Fructose, in semen, 15
FSH. See Follicle stimulating hormone
  (FSH)

Gamete intrafallopian transfer (GIFT)
  clinical development of, 126
  cost of, 128
  current clinical results of, 128–132
  experimental background of, 125–126
  future improvements in, 137–139
  indications and patient requirements
    for, 126–127
  vs. IVF-ET, 127–128
  for male factor infertility, 131–132
  outside IVF laboratory, 133
  technique of, 133–137
  for unexplained infertility, 131
Gamete loading, for GIFT, 135
Genetic disorders, 10–11
Glycerol, for cryopreservation, 142, 144–
  145, 147
Gonadotropin(s). See also Human cho-
    rionic gonadotropin (hCG); Human
    menopausal gonadotropin (hMG,
    Pergonal)
  in ovulation induction, 61–62, 66–67
  regimens for, 79–81
Gonadotropin releasing hormone (GnRH),
    hypothalamic-pituitary influence on,
    61–62
Gonadotropin releasing hormone (GnRH)
    analogs
  follicular development with, 73
  with hMG, 81–85
  in ovulation induction, 67
  protocol for, 83–85
Graafian follicle, 62
Gynogenesis, 121

Ham's F-10, 104
Hamster test, 16, 21–22
Hemizona assay (HZA), 23
hFSH (urinary FSH), 45, 81, 85
History, psychosocial, 33, 34
House Bill No. 1660, 173–176
Human chorionic gonadotropin (hCG)
  dosage and timing of, 45, 78–79
  and estradiol level, 74–75
  for luteal phase deficiency, 86
  in ovulation induction, 66–67, 78–79
  sonography after, 74
Human menopausal gonadotropin (hMG,
    Pergonal)
  with clomiphene citrate, 79
  dosage and timing of, 45, 79–81
  and estradiol level, 74

follicular maturation with, 70, 73
GnRH analog with, 81–85
LH surge with, 76–77
in ovulation induction, 66–67
sensitivity to, 80
Hypogonadotropic hypogonadism, 81
Hypothalamus, in ovulation induction, 61–62, 81
HZA (hemizona assay), 23

Idiopathic infertility, 8–9
GIFT for, 9, 131
IVF for, 9–10
Immunologic factor infertility, 8, 15–16, 20–21
Implantation, description of, 50
Indications, 3
cervical factor, 8
endometriosis, 5–7
genetic disorders, 10–11
idiopathic infertility, 8–10
immunologic factor, 8
male factor, 7–8
ovarian disorders, 10
patient age, 10
tubal disease, 3–5
uterine disease, 11
Induction of ovulation. See Ovulation induction
Informed consent, 51–58
Inhibin, in follicular development, 76
Injections, 41, 45
Insurance coverage
Blue Cross/Blue Shield policy on, 165
legislation on, 168–176
physicians' support for, 166–167
Interview, 33, 41
Intrauterine insemination (IUI), 125, 132, 155–156
IVF program
acceptance into, 28
description of, 49–50
IVF team, 39–42

Justice, 152

Kallmann's syndrome, 61

Laboratory preparation
culture medium in, 104
equipment for, 112
for oocyte retrieval, 106–111
organization and quality control in, 103
protein supplements in, 104
of semen, 105–106, 107
supplies for, 112–113
Laparoscopy
gamete intrafallopian transfer by, 135–137
oocyte retrieval by, 92, 93–94, 95, 106
Legislation, 159, 168–176
Leukocytes, in semen, 15
Leuprolide acetate (Lupron)
dosage of, 45
with hMG therapy, 81–85

Luteal phase deficiency, 67, 79–80
Luteal phase support
for GIFT, 137
for IVF, 86–87
Luteinizing hormone (LH)
in dominance of follicle, 70
with GnRH analog, 81, 82, 83, 84
hypothalamic-pituitary influence on, 61–62
in intraovarian follicular regulation, 62
in ovulation, 65
in ovulation induction, 66–67
in recruitment of follicle, 63
spontaneous surge of, 70, 76–77
in two-cell theory, 80
Luteinizing hormone (LHRH) releasing hormone, hypothalamic-pituitary influence on, 61–62

Male factor infertility
diagnosis of, 14–16
donor insemination for, 155
GIFT for, 131–132
as indication, 7–8
IVF for, 16–21
laboratory evaluation of, 21–23
laboratory preparation for, 23–24
new techniques for, 24
prognosis for, 21–23
success rate with, 6, 8
treatment of, 16
MAST (Michigan Alcohol Screening Test), 35
Medical Research Council of Great Britain, on ethical principles, 159–160
Menotropins. See Human menopausal gonadotropin (hMG, Pergonal)
Mental status examination, 33
Metrodin (urinary FSH), 45, 81, 85
Michigan Alcohol Screening Test (MAST), 35
Microinjection, of sperm, 24
Minicool freezing machine, 145
Miscarriage. See Spontaneous abortion
Morula, 116
Multiple gestations
with GIFT, 130
with IVF, 55, 67

NEO Personality Inventory (NEO-PI), 34–35
Nonmaleficence, 152
Nurse coordinator, 39–42, 43

Office procedure, 43–50
Oligospermia
GIFT for, 127, 131–132
IVF for, 8, 16–18, 19
Oocyte
abnormal, 119, 121
abnormal fertilization of, 119–121
cleavage of, 116–119
donor, 156, 157
at fertilization, 115–116, 117
before fertilization, 114–115

Oocyte—*Continued*
  maturation of, 114–115
  primary, 114
  polyspermic, 121
  secondary, 114
Oocyte donation, ethics of, 156, 157
Oocyte preparation, for GIFT, 134
Oocyte retrieval
  consent form for, 51, 55–56
  data sheet for, 108
  description of, 49
  description sheet for, 109
  for GIFT, 134
  IVF team during, 41
  laboratory procedure for, 106–111
  laparoscopic, 92, 93–94, 95, 106
  psychological issues with, 28
  sonographic, 92–93, 94–97, 106
Oogonia, 114
Oral contraceptives, programmed cycles
    with, 81
Ovarian cyst, 71
Ovarian disorders, 10
Ovarian hyperstimulation
  aims of, 69
  CC/hMG in, 79–81
  clinical parameters of, 76
  estrogen measurement with, 74–76
  GnRH analog/hMG therapy in, 81–85
  hCG administration in, 78–79
  luteal phase support in, 86–87
  methods of controlled, 79
  oral contraceptives in, 81
  sonography of, 71–74
  spontaneous LH surge in, 76–77
Ovarian hyperstimulation syndrome
  estradiol level and, 67, 76
  factors predictive of, 85–86
  hCG and, 67
  incidence of, 85
  minimizing risk of, 67
  pathophysiologic mechanisms of, 86
  presentation of, 85
  risk of, 51, 54, 55
  treatment of, 86
Ovulation, 65
Ovulation induction
  clomiphene citrate in, 66
  complications of, 67–68
  consent forms for, 51, 54–55
  corpus luteum formation in, 65
  dominance in, 64–65
  for GIFT, 133–134
  human gonadotropin therapy in, 66–67
  hypothalamic-pituitary influence on,
    61–62
  intraovarian follicular regulation in,
    62–65, 70, 72
  IVF team during, 41
  ovulation in, 65
  physiologic principles of, 61–68
  psychological issues with, 28
  recruitment of follicle in, 62–63
  selection of follicle in, 63–64

Parthenogenesis, 121
Patient selection. *See* Indications
Percoll gradient technique, 23–24
Pergonal. *See* Human menopausal gonado-
    tropin (hMG, Pergonal)
Personality Inventory, 34–35
Personnel, 39–42
Pituitary, in ovulation induction, 61–62,
    81
Planar freezing machine, 145
PLISSIT, 30–32
Polar body, 114
Polyspermy, 121
Postcoital test, 15–16
Postoperative instructions, 47
Precycle, IVF team during, 39
Pre-embryo donation, ethics of, 156–157
Prefreeze stage, 143
Preovulatory follicle, 62
Progesterone
  consent form for injections of, 56
  in corpus luteum formation, 65
  dosage of, 45
  with GnRH analog, 82, 83, 84
  for luteal phase deficiency, 86–87
Pronuclear stage, cryopreservation of, 148
Pronuclear stage tubal transfer (PROST),
    138
Pronuclei, multiple, 121
Propanediol, for cryopreservation, 144,
    148
Protein supplements, preparation of, 104
Protocol, 45–48
Psychological evaluation, 32–34
Psychological intervention, 30–32
Psychological issues, during IVF, 27–30,
    31
Psychometric evaluation, 34–35
Psychosocial history, 33, 34

Quality control, in laboratory areas, 103

Rapid freezing, 144
Reconstructive tubal surgery, vs. IVF-ET,
    163
Recruitment, of follicle, 62–63, 69, 70
Repeated IVF attempts, psychological is-
    sues with, 29

Schedule, 45–46
Secretary, 43
Seeding, in cryopreservation, 143
Selection, of follicle, 63–64, 69, 70, 72
Semen analysis, 14–15, 105
Semen collection, protocol for, 47–48,
    105–106
Semen preparation, 105–106, 107
Senate Bill No. 793, 168–172
Serophene. *See* Clomiphene citrate (CC,
    Clomid, Serophene)
Serum supplements, preparation of, 104
Sexually transmitted diseases, in artificial
    donor insemination, 156
Slippery-slope concept, 153–155

Slow freezing, 143–144
Sonography
    description for patients of, 46
    of follicular development, 71–74
    in oocyte retrieval, 92–93, 94–97, 106
SPA (sperm penetration assay), 21–22
Sperm agglutination tests, 16
Sperm antibodies, 8, 15–16, 20–21
Sperm concentration, 8, 15, 16–18, 19
Sperm donation, ethics of, 155–156
Sperm immobilization test, 16
Sperm immunobead test, 16
Sperm morphology, 20
Sperm motility, 15, 18–20
Sperm penetration assay (SPA), 21–22
Sperm preparation
    for GIFT, 134
    for IVF, 23–24
Spontaneous abortion
    vs. general population, 167
    with GIFT, 131
    with ovulation induction, 67, 74, 83
Staff, 39–42
Staff burnout, 35
Success rates
    on consent form, 55
    per cycle, 3, 167
    by diagnosis, 6
    with endometriosis, 6, 7
    for GIFT, 128–132
    with male factor infertility, 6, 8
    and number of embryos transferred, 98–
        99
    with tubal disease, 4–5, 6

Sucrose, in cryopreservation, 145, 148
Support group, 31
Surrogacy, ethics of, 158–159
Swim-up method, 23

Termination of IVF, psychological issues
    with, 29–30
Thawing phase, 144
Thawing solutions, 147, 148
Tubal disease, 3–4
    success rates with, 4–5, 6
Tubal reanastomosis, 4
Two-cell theory, 62, 80

Unexplained infertility, 8–9
    GIFT for, 9, 131
    IVF for, 9–10
Urinary FSH (hFSH, Metrodin), 45, 81, 85
Uterine disease, 11

Vasectomy, 16
Vitrification, 144

Waiting list, 39, 43

Zona drilling, 24
Zona-free hamster test, 16, 21–22
Zona pellucida, 114, 115
    fractured or empty, 119, 120
Zygote intrafallopian transfer, 138